OXFORD MEDICAL PUBLICATIONS

Hospital Infection Control

Hospital Infection Control
Setting up with minimal resources

SHAHEEN MEHTAR

Consultant Microbiologist,
North Middlesex Hospital
and
Senior Lecturer (Hon.), Royal Free Hospital

Oxford   New York   Tokyo
OXFORD UNIVERSITY PRESS
1992

Oxford University Press, Walton Street, Oxford OX2 6DP
Oxford   New York   Toronto
Delhi   Bombay   Calcutta   Madras   Karachi
Kuala Lumpur   Singapore   Hong Kong   Tokyo
Nairobi   Dar es Salaam   Cape Town
Melbourne   Auckland   Madrid
and associated companies in
Berlin   Ibadan

Oxford is a trade mark of Oxford University Press

Published in the United States
by Oxford University Press Inc., New York

A catalogue record for this book is available from the British Library

Library of Congress Cataloging in Publication Data
(Data available on request)

ISBN 0-19-262266-8 (hb)
ISBN 0-19-262033-9 (pb)

Typeset by
Footnote Graphics, Warminster, Wilts
Printed in Great Britain by
Biddles Ltd., Guildford & King's Lynn

To the home team

Acknowledgements

I am deeply grateful to Janice Stenning, for her help in typing the manuscript, and to Eric Taylor for his advice and laborious editing.

Foreword

Graham A. J. Ayliffe
Emeritus Professor of Medical Microbiology,
formerly Director of the Hospital Infection Research Laboratory,
Birmingham,
and Chairman of the International Federation of Infection Control

The spread of infection is a major problem in developing countries but the principles of effective control are the same throughout the world. However, alternative methods are sometimes necessary due to a lack of resources, such as clean water, electricity, or disposables. Recommendations for control of infection in the industrial countries are often not based on good evidence, and simpler methods can be equally effective; for example, clinical waste (apart from syringe needles) represents a minimal infection hazard, and provided it is handled and stored safely, does not require incineration as a control of infection measure. A return to the production of reprocessible items such as syringes and gloves may also be worthwhile in the absence of reliable supplies of single-use items. The uncontrolled use of antibiotics leads to the emergence of resistant bacterial strains, and the resultant requirement for new antibiotics can considerably increase the cost of infection control. The rapid spread of HIV infection in some countries has also emphasized the need for good infection control techniques.

Dr Shaheen Mehtar has used her wide experience in the UK and developing countries to deal with these problems. She has written a useful book in which both the optimal and possible alternative methods are described. Information on administrative aspects, modes of spread, and costs of infection policies and guidelines are concisely presented, and practical details are included where necessary. As Dr Mehtar states in the preface, control of infection need not be expensive. Handwashing at the right time and using a correct technique remains the cornerstone of prevention of spread of infection, but good training of medical and nursing staff in safe control of infection techniques is essential.

This book fills an important gap and can be recommended to anyone wishing to set up a hospital infection control programme, but should be particularly useful in countries with minimal resources.

Preface

Hospital-acquired infection (nosocomial infection) is a world-wide problem. The widespread use of antibiotics and advances in hospital practice have resulted in an increased incidence and recognition of nosocomial infection, which can be caused by antibiotic-resistant Gram-positive and Gram-negative bacteria.

There is a misconception that infection control programmes are expensive and therefore beyond the reach of most hospitals. In fact, the opposite is true. Infection control is based on common sense and safe practice, and a well-balanced infection control programme should save the hospital a considerable amount of money. For example, an outbreak of Gram-negative bacilli can be controlled effectively by meticulous hand hygiene and heat disinfection of equipment, rather than by prescribing expensive antibiotics, which may further contribute to the problem.

The principles of the control of nosocomial infection are the same throughout the world, but richer countries use more sophisticated methods to monitor and predict outbreaks. In the UK, each problem is dealt with vigorously on a day-to-day basis to minimize the spread of nosocomial pathogens; we believe that this system proves more economic in the long run.

This book is written mainly for infection-control doctors and nurses, and for committees setting up infection control programmes. It covers the application in practice of essential principles of infection control, and appropriate alternatives for countries with minimal resources. It should therefore provide a useful reference for those setting up a sound and workable infection control programme.

London   S.M.
April 1992

Contents

Abbreviations

BS	British Standard
HBV	Hepatitis B virus
HEPA	High efficiency particulate air filter
HIV	Human immunodeficiency virus
IC	Infection control
MRSA	Methicillin-resistant *Staphylococcus aureus*
TWA	Time weighed average
AHU	Air handling unit
MRGN	Multiply antibiotic-resistant Gram-negative
i.v.	Intravenous
i.m.	Intramuscular
CVP	Central venous pressure line
ICC	Infection control committee
ITU	Intensive therapy unit
Md	Mega dalton
SSD	Sterile services department
RTI	Respiratory tract infection
EEC	European Economic Community
High Risk	Specimens taken from patients with known or suspected transferable infection
TSSU	Theatre sterile services unit
BCP	Bacteria carrying particles
p.p.m.	Parts per million
OHD	Occupational health department
H and S	Health and Safety
COSHH	Control of Substances Hazardous to Health

Part 1
The infection control policy

1. Nosocomial pathogens

Nosocomial pathogens (alert organisms) are bacteria or viruses that cause or spread hospital outbreaks. The Infection Control (IC) team must investigate every occurrence of nosocomial infection. Nosocomial pathogens may arise, *de novo*, in a hospital unit or be brought in by staff or patients admitted to the hospital. They include:

- Pathogens not isolated on the affected unit before, e.g.:
  —*Staphylococcus aureus*;
  —*Salmonella* species;
  —*Pseudomonas aeruginosa*;
  —rotavirus;
  —group A streptococci.
- Pathogens arising in response to changes in antibiotic sensitivity, e.g.:
  —methicillin-resistant *Staphylococcus aureus* (MRSA);
  —gentamicin-resistant Gram-negative bacilli in patients with urinary catheters.
- Pathogens previously isolated but now causing a new clinical problem, e.g.:
  —coagulase-negative staphylococci isolated from central venous lines;
  —*Pseudomonas* species isolated from ventilator tubing and equipment.
- 'New' pathogens, i.e. those previously considered to be commensals or of low pathogenicity, e.g.:
  —*Serratia marcenscens*;
  —*Enterococcus faecalis*;
  —*Candida albicans* and other fungi.

It may take time to establish or recognize a particular pathogen responsible for a nosocomial infection and, during this time, surveillance data are helpful to demonstrate clustering of cases and to warn the IC team of potential cross-infection or of new outbreaks.

The spread of nosocomial pathogens

The two main routes of transmission are by contact (either direct or indirect) and by air-borne spread.

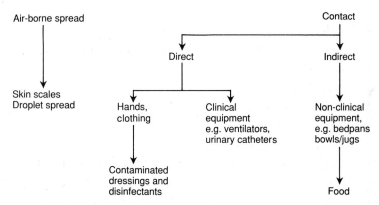

Fig. 1.1 Method of spread.

Contact

Direct contact

Direct contact results in contamination of a previously uninfected patient:

- by the hospital staff (doctors and nurses);
- from bedclothes and personal items;
- via the hands—the most common means of spreading nosocomial pathogens.

Indirect contact

Indirect contact is less common and arises from:

- Clinical equipment that has not been properly disinfected or sterilized.
- Shared non-clinical equipment (e.g. bedpans and bowls).
- Transmission of multiply antibiotic-resistant organisms from the kitchens and utensils.

- Disinfectants contaminated with bacteria.
- Sluice rooms (splash contamination).
- Inadequately sterilized dressings.
- Re-use of inadequately sterilized disposable items (e.g. needles and syringes—this practice should not be allowed, see p. 40).

Air-borne spread

Air-borne spread is less common than spread by direct or indirect contact. However, it can occur:

- by droplet spread;
- by air currents transporting skin scales from infected burns or dermatitis patients;
- when shaking out bed clothing;
- in busy units with a lot of movement of staff between beds.

Table 1.1 summarizes the routes of transmission of nosocomial pathogens.

Why do nosocomial infections arise?

There are many reasons for the spread of nosocomial infections in hospital, including:

Table 1.1 Nosocomial pathogens

Organism	Carriage site	Method of spread
Staphylococcus aureus	Nose, groin hairline, skin lesions, wounds, urinary catheters	Hands, skin scales, droplet spread
Group A streptococci	Anterior nares, throat, skin lesions, wounds	Hands, skin
Gram-negative bacilli: Multiply antibiotic-resistant *Pseudomonas aeruginosa*	Stool, urine, moist skin lesions	Hands, urinary catheter, non-clinical equipment, ventilators, disinfectants, moist areas in the environment

- Lowered immunity—most patients have reduced immunity to infection.
- Overcrowding.
- Inadequate facilities.
- The use of untrained relatives as patient attendants (resulting in less than ideal care as far as cleanliness is concerned).
- Poor design and planning of hospitals.
- Referral from other hospitals where there may be an endemic problem.
- Transfer to or from specialized hospitals or units with a high usage of antibiotics (e.g. burns and oncology units). Such patients carry bacteria that are often resistant to the antibiotics that combat these infections.
- Admission of carriers for unrelated medical conditions (e.g. a Salmonella carrier admitted to a surgical ward).
- Under-staffing, which can result in a breakdown of procedure and to short-cuts.
- Transfer of medical practitioners from one unit to another or between hospitals.

Factors increasing the risk of hospital-acquired infection

Many factors increase the risk of a hospital-acquired infection:

- Patient risk factors:
  —extremes of ages (i.e. premature babies, elderly patients);
  —immunocompromised patients;
  —concurrent disease (e.g. diabetes);
  —chemotherapy;
  —steroid therapy;
  —antibiotic therapy (causing resistance);
  —intravenous therapy;
  —urinary catheterization;
  —surgical procedures, particularly when:
    * skin disinfection is inadequate;
    * the patient is subject to long periods of anaesthesia (which impair respiratory defences);
    * the patients is being given a prosthesic implant.

—respiratory ventilation;
—long hospital stay;

- Environmental risk factors via direct or indirect contact:
  —prolonged hospitalization (increases nosocomial infection rates);
  —specialized areas with specialized bacteria (antibiotic-resistant plasmids);
  —disinfectants (colonized with multiply antibiotic-resistant bacteria)
  —sterile services;   ⎫
  —non-clinical equipment;   ⎪ These may be
  —water supply (developing countries); ⎬ or may become
  —food supply and kitchens. ⎭ contaminated.

- Nature of the organism:
  —high virulence (e.g. *Staphylococcus aureus*, Group A streptococci);
  —opportunism secondary to antibiotic therapy and lower body defences;
  —colonization—post-instrumentation;
  —invasion secondary to viral infection;
  —high infecting dose (i.e. 10^6 organisms/millilitre).

Summary

- Every outbreak of hospital-acquired infection must be investigated by the IC team.
- Nosocomial infections are caused by:
  —pathogens that have not been isolated on the ward/unit before;
  —altered antibiotic sensitivity;
  —known pathogens that did not pose a clinical problem in the past;
  —'new' pathogens.
- Nosocomial pathogens are spread by:
  —contact (direct and indirect);
  —air (droplet spread, air currents).
- There are three main types of risk factor:
  —patient risk factors;
  —environmental risk factors;
  —risk factors relating to the character of the infection organism.

2. Infection control and management structure

The economics of an infection control programme

The Cooke report (1988) recommends that every hospital in the UK should have an Infection Control (IC) team. However, in other, developing, countries infection control is in its infancy and often relies on the goodwill of staff. Unfortunately, infection control programmes in these countries are often given little credibility, although effective control measures have been found to save hospitals significant amounts of money and are therefore vital for economic, as well as for patient health, reasons.

A study by Currie and Maynard (1989) costed hospital-acquired infection in England at £115 million in 1987, and suggested that £36 million of this could be avoided by more effective infection control measures. This would, in theory, release funds for redeployment elsewhere in the health service.

Thus, although effective infection control policies require substantial support in their initial stages (both financially and administratively), these initial costs should be compared with the long-term savings of effective infection control.

The costs of hospital-acquired infection

Although much has been written about nosocomial infection rates, an acceptable rate of infection has not yet been established. There is clearly a risk of acquiring infection whilst in hospital, but the degree of risk depends upon the category of patient.

Specific costs of hospital-acquired infection

The rates of infection after intravenous therapy are known to vary from 2 to 25 per cent, with a bacteraemia rate of 1 to 10 per cent for peripheral lines (Maki 1989) and between 4 and 20 per cent for central and hyperalimentation lines (Mehtar 1982). An estimated

10–12 million i.v. cannulae are sold in the UK per year so a 1 per cent incidence of bacteraemia (Macfarlane et al. 1981) results in 100 000 bacteraemic episodes per year. If only 50 per cent of these require antibiotics for a minimum of five days then the cost, at £4 per day, would be £1 000 000 (50 000 patients × 5 days of antibiotic treatment = 250 000 patient treatment days, at £4 per day), and this is probably a conservative estimate.

A 1-day prevalence survey of UK hospitals (Report on the National Survey of Infection in Hospital, 1981) showed that urinary tract infections represented 22 per cent of hospital infections and that 33.3 per cent were hospital-acquired; 21.2 per cent of these infections were in catheterized patients. The bacterial acquisition rate with a closed system of urinary drainage is 5–10 per cent per catheterized day; with an open system it is 100 per cent in 4 days (Bisno and Waldvogel 1989). This represents an enormous cost in terms of bed days, antibiotics, and medical care.

Sacks and McGowan (1981) have showed that nosocomial infections can prolong hospital stay by up to 13.3 days—this is twice as long as a normal stay. In addition, the cost of antibiotics (usually parenteral), dressings and nursing time must be considered. The cost of a 5-day hospital stay of a patient requiring parenteral antibiotic therapy at the author's hospital is given in Table 2.1.

Table 2.1 Costs of a 5-day hospital stay for an infected patient requiring parenteral antibiotic therapy (North Middlesex Hospital, 1991)

Item	Cost per day(£)	Cost for 5 days
Basic cost per patient	140	700
hotel expenses, bed, food, linen, electricity, etc		
Intravenous antibiotics	115	600
pharmacy costs (4 doses)	66	
reconstitute drug (16.50 per dose)		
includes fluids, minibags, labour		
administration sets, cannulae, etc	12	
cost of antibiotic(s)	37	
Protective clothing and hand		40
disinfection		
Disposables (e.g. clothing, equipment)		15
TOTAL COST		1355

This cost does not include manpower or laboratory tests, as these vary and therefore cannot be included in a general estimate.

Outbreaks of infection are expensive and are a great drain on the resources of the hospital. For example, the costs of a 5-week outbreak of methicillin-resistant *Staphylococcus aureus* (MRSA) involving seven ITU wards, 36 patients, and necessitating the screening of 2245 patients and staff are shown in Table 2.2.

Table 2.1 The cost of a 5-week outbreak of MRSA

Item and usage	Cost (£)	Total for 5 weeks (£)
ITU and ward screening (2245 patients were screened)	0.65	1459.25
bacteriology swab (× 2)		
culture media (agar plates and broth)		
Antibiotics		
mupirocin (30 patients × 2 tubes)	4.00/tube	240.00
vancomycin (12 patients; 161 treatment days)	40/day	6440.00
Disinfectants		
Hibisol (per 500 ml)	1.50	20.00
Hibiscrub (per 5 ml)	1.50	15.00
Protective clothing (2 boxes/rolls per ward; 5 wards)		
gloves (plastic; per 100)	3.45	160.00
gloves (latex; per 100)	8.90	400.00
masks (per 300)	17.50	150.00
aprons (per 1000)	25.75	550.00
Cleaning		
terminal clean	400/ward	2000.00
domestic cleaning (per session)	125/ward	1500.00
TOTAL COSTS		12,935.00

In 1984, an outbreak of hospital-acquired infection caused by a multiply antibiotic-resistant plasmid (98 Md) affected all species of Gram-negative bacilli in the author's hospital (the North Middlesex Hospital, London). The outbreak involved 520 patients over a period of 27 months and necessitated establishing a 20-cubicle isolation ward for 6 weeks. The total costs involved for this isolation ward, including the laboratory costs, were compared to the costs of a ward matched for age and patient type over the same (6-week) period. The isolation ward cost £36 000 more; Table 2.3).

Table 2.3 Comparison of costs for a 20-bedded isolation ward and a non-infected ward during an outbreak of multiple antibiotic-resistant plasmid (the North Middlesex Hospital, 1983)

Item Cost/item (£)	Usage/week	Cost	Cost/6 weeks (£)
Non-infected ward			
Protective clothing			
aprons	4 rolls	19.49 (100/roll)	467.76
gloves	4 boxes	2.18 (per box)	52.32
Disinfectants			
chlorhexidine			
hand-wash	750 ml	1.50 (per 500 ml)	13.50
alcohol rub	750 ml	1.75 (per 500 ml)	15.72
phenolic	none used		
Nursing			
specialized	37 hours	76.00 (per week)	456.00
Laundry		50.00 (per week)	300.00
Infected ward			
Protective clothing			
aprons	20 rolls	19.49 (per 100)	2338.00
gloves	20 boxes	2.18 (per box)	261.60
Disinfectants			
chlorhexidine			
hand-wash	500 ml × 20	1.50 (per 500 ml)	
alcohol rub	500 ml × 20	1.75 (per 500 ml)	390.00
phenolic	300 litres	1.30 (per litre)	2340.00
Nursing (extra)	19 FTE	4.60 (per hour)	19,600.00
Laundry (extra)		50.00 (per week)	300.00
Domestics (2 full time)	76 hours/week	1.64/hour	1500.00
Terminal cleaning	90 sessions	20.00 (per session)	1800.00
Screening (microbiology)			9200.00
TOTAL			37,729.60

FTE, full-time equivalents.

The cost of establishing an infection control programme

The costs of establishing the major portion of an infection control programme (90 per cent) is minimal; the cost of attaining one hundred percent is much higher (Fig. 2.1). It is therefore prudent to start with programme designed to achieve the first 90 per cent and gradually to build up to the final 10 per cent as revenue savings are realized.

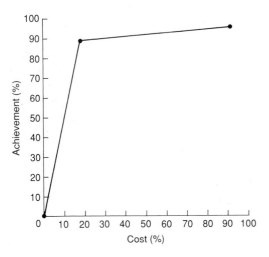

Fig. 2.1 Graphic representation of achievable infection control programme versus cost.

The costs involved in setting up an infection control programme include:

- Predictable costs:
    —staff costs—IC nurse, secretarial, and administrative plus training and education;
    —protective clothing;
    —monitoring equipment;
    —data surveillance equipment—including a computer system and software;
    —maintenance of equipment;
    —laboratory tests for routine monitoring of specialized areas;
    —pre-employment screening and immunization.
- Unpredictable costs:
    —costs for individual infective patient episodes;
    —outbreaks that cannot be forecast.

Staff costs

Staff costs depend entirely on the number of staff dedicated to infection control.

In hospitals in the UK, the Infection Control (IC) doctor is usually a clinical microbiologist and therefore is not an additional expense. However, in countries where infection control practitioners are separate entities, there *will* be an additional expense.

The infection control nurses are full-time and will fall within the IC budget. To be effective they must be available to staff throughout the hospital at all times, and so radiopagers, telephones and administrative help are necessary. Smaller units in the UK (up to 500 beds) usually have one IC nurse; larger units have two (or more) (Table 2.4).

Table 2.4 Approximate cost of setting up an IC programme in the UK (1991)

Item	Cost (£)
Senior IC nurse	22,000
Secretarial help	11,000
Training and education of IC nurses	2,000–3,000
Monitoring equipment	2,000–3,000
Laboratory reagents	500–1,000
Stand alone computer system (for data surveillance)	3,000
Software	500
TOTAL COST	44,000

Costs will differ in each country.

Equipment

Equipment to monitor nosocomial infections, for example an air sampler, is not expensive, although it requires regular maintenance, which must also be included in the IC budget (Table 2.5).

Surveillance data collection

Surveillance by the IC team is necessary to monitor outbreaks and for forecasting new outbreaks. Although this may be done manually, a computer system is more effective and will repay its initial expense.

Table 2.5 Relative costs of achieving 90 to 99.9 per cent infection control

To achieve 90 per cent infection control		To achieve 99.9 per cent infection control (the last 10 per cent of control is much more expensive)
Saves money	Minimal cost	
Disinfectant policy	Recycling protective clothing	Bedpan disinfectors
Antibiotic policy	Manual data collection	Establishing a Sterile Services Department
Waste disposal policy	Education and training	Incineration facilities
	Reorganization into special units	Upgrading the water supply
		Upgrading the operating theatres
		Using disposable protective clothing
		Computerization of data collection

False economy

There seems to be a widespread belief that money can be saved by recycling items of disposable equipment. This view is short-sighted when one considers to amount of money spent on antibiotics to treat patients infected by inadequately sterilized equipment (and also when the cost of sterilizing this equipment is calculated).

However, recycling gloves for sterile and non-sterile procedures is cost-effective when sterilization is effective—the reuse of gloves with alcohol rub between patients has also been shown to cost-effective.

Cost benefit of infection control programmes

The implementation of infection control policies can result in considerable cost savings. Table 2.6 shows a few examples from the North Middlesex Hospital.

The benefits of infection control programmes are best shown by a baseline assessment of infection rates, procedures and practice for 6 months prior to the introduction of an infection control programme and identical monitoring for the first 6 months of the programme

Table 2.6 Examples of cost savings resulting from infection control policies over a 10-year period (1980–1990)

Item	Saving (£)
Antibiotic rationalization (establishing	50,000
principles for antibiotic use)	
24-hour prophylaxis	
7-day treatment then review	
stopping antibiotics when they are not needed	
restricted topical antibiotics	
restricted reporting	
treatment by junior staff, with senior staff available to give advice	
Disinfectant policy	15,000
no routine environmental disinfection	
hand disinfection policy	
no soaking of instruments (except fibre optics)	
Rationalization of disposable equipment	5,000
one type of general-use cannula only	
one type of administration set for blood and one for solutions	
reduce bandages and dressing to one of each type	
use correct gauge and duration urinary catheters	
establish policy of usage of sterile and non-sterile gloves	
Topping up ward stock (1800 per ward × 5 wards/year)	9,000
Centralization of sterile services	10,000
TOTAL RECURRING SAVINGS	90,000

Item	Capital expenditure (£)
Total savings per year	90,000
Expenditure	
autoclaves (× 2)	32,000
bedpan disinfectors (× 6)	21,000
ventilator circuits	10,000
Total expenditure	63,000
SAVINGS PER ANNUM:	90,000 − 63,000 = 22,000
REDEPLOYMENT OF SAVINGS	
Further expected purchases	
fume cabinet for glutaraldehyde extraction	3,000
closed circuit endoscopy disinfector	7,000
upgrading bedpan disinfectors	3,000

and a further 6 months monitoring once the programme is established and understood. This exercise is very worthwhile to demonstrate to the administrators (and other clinical colleagues) just how effective an IC programme can be.

3. The infection control committee

The role of the infection control committee

The role of the Infection Control Committee (ICC) is to:

- Formulate and monitor patient-care policies.
- Advise on the purchase of clinical and non-clinical equipment (as this may be involved, directly or indirectly, in cross-infection).
- Liaise with nursing and medical staff on new policies and procedures.
- Educate all hospital staff in the infection control programme.
- Realize savings resulting from the infection control programme and redeploy these funds to improve patient care.
- Take part in medical audit, as well as being subject to medical audit itself.

Membership of the ICC

The ICC should be made up of:

- infection control doctor;
- infection control nurse(s); these members form the IC team (see p. 20)
- administrator;
- representative of the medical staff;
- representative of the nursing staff;
- pharmacist;
- engineer;
- sterile supplies manager.

Infection control doctor

This should be a medically qualified person who is interested in, and who spends the majority of his/her time involved in, hospital infection control. In the UK this person is usually a clinical micro-biologist, but could be an infectious diseases physician, a surgeon or any other medical person whose opinion is respected, who has knowledge of nosocomial infection and who is willing to give sufficient time to the role.

The infection control doctor must:

- establish a close working relationship with all medical and non-medical hospital staff;
- should always be available to advise on all aspects of infection control.

It is practical, although not always possible, for this person to chair the ICC.

Infection control nurse(s)

The infection control nurses should be trained in the clinical aspects of all hospital practice, particularly in the high risk areas, e.g. operating theatres, intensive care units and neonatal units. They should work closely with the IC doctor and with the nursing staff. They are responsible for:

- furthering the infection control policy by educating nursing staff;
- suggesting changes to nursing practice and ward procedures;
- collection of surveillance data;
- helping to implement infection control policies;
- research.

Hospital staff must have confidence in the infection control nurses if they are to refer to them for advice.

Medical staff representative

This person is usually a surgeon or physician who is concerned with problems in infection and can bring medical expertise to the committee. They are another link with the medical staff and with areas of clinical practice and should advise the ICC on recent advances in medical procedures that may have infection control implications.

Pharmacist

Recommendations made by the ICC on antibiotic and disinfectant policies are channelled via the hospital Pharmacy Department. The Pharmacist should advise staff on the appropriate use of disinfectants and keep records of cost and usage of antibiotics and disinfectants. These records should be presented to the ICC on a regular basis.

Nursing representative

This should be a senior member of the nursing administration and education department. The role of the nursing representative is:

- to convey the recommendations of the ICC to the nursing staff;
- to ensure that the nurse education programme includes IC policies and procedures.

There should be close links with the nurse training department, if one exists (if not, a training programme should be started). The nursing representative is responsible for feedback to the ICC on IC policy-related problems that occur on the wards.

Engineer

The engineer is an essential part of the ICC. Every hospital would be well advised to employ an engineer—the costs savings in real terms are considerable. The engineer should:

- test and maintain equipment associated with the infection control programme (e.g. bedpan disinfectors, autoclaves, incinerators);
- monitor and maintain the water and electricity supplies;
- install and/or repair existing equipment to meet required standards.

The hospital engineers should always be consulted before any new equipment is purchased, to ensure that it follows hospital policies on maintenance and servicing. The IC team should be consulted for advice on sterilization and disinfection of equipment.

Sterile supplies manager

The manager of the Sterile Services Department is an essential member of the ICC. They need to work closely with the IC team and the Engineering Department and must have a working know-ledge of safe methods of disinfection and sterilization and be able to advise on quality assurance and safe practices.

Administrator

The administrator may have a medical background and is respons-ible for ensuring that the recommendations and policies of the ICC are widely distributed and implemented in the hospital. They may also be responsible for the finances, ensuring that savings resulting from the infection control policy are rechannelled into further developments in infection control and improved patient care.

The above are essential members of the ICC. **Co-opted members** may include a:

- representative from the domestic department;
- representative from the catering department;
- porters' representative;
- junior doctors' representative;
- representative from the anaesthetic department;
- operating theatre representative;
- medical supplies and purchasing representative;
- representative from the occupational health department;
- health and safety representative.

The ICC is thus made up of members of the hospital staff who are involved with day-to-day patient care, are active, concerned, and well-respected.

The infection control team

The IC team, which comprises the IC doctor, the IC nurse, the administrator, and occasionally a medical technician, is the core of the ICC. It should:

- Advise and educate staff on all aspects of infection control.
- Improve and monitor the safe practices of patient care (being careful not to take away clinical freedom or to undertake direct management of the patients).

- Give advice on:
  —the sterilization of new clinical equipment;
  —the protection of patients and staff;
  —the safe handling of clinical waste;
  —planning and building.

It should work at ward level, producing policies, procedures, and recommendations to improve standards. These policies should then be forwarded to the ICC for deliberation and comment (Fig. 3.1). When drawing up a policy, the IC Team should:

- Consider whether the present system is satisfactory. If yes, point out the potential problems relating to infection control. If no, would the staff support a different policy?

- Consider how the new policy will affect present practice.

- Meet all the departments concerned and discuss the policy. Any unacceptable aspects should be modified as required.

- Present the policy to the ICC for approval and authorization by the hospital administration.

- Identify a contact person (usually a member of the IC team) who will advise and clarify queries on the policy.

- Circulate the policy throughout the hospital.

- Add the policy to the IC manual.

In some countries it may be more politically astute to have a two-tier system. The administrators (Medical Superintendent) and

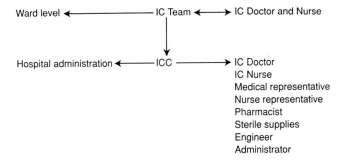

Fig. 3.1 Working relationship of the IC team with the rest of the hospital.

Heads of Department make up the Management of Infection Committee (MIC) and the Infection Control (working) personnel form the IC Committee. Policies are then passed from the ICC to the MIC for approval.

Hospital planning

Ideally, the IC team should be involved in the planning of the hospital before it is built, and should always be involved in planning any structural alterations to the hospital and in the development of any specialized department. It may notice potential problems related to infection control and, by advising at the planning stage, may reduce future outbreaks of infection.

The IC manual

The IC manual constitutes the infection control practice of the hospital and is a useful tool for ward-level teaching and education of all staff—medical and non-medical. It provides uniformity and standardization of patient care and staff practice.

When the IC policies have been agreed, the administrator should present them to the Executive Board of the hospital, or equivalent, for approval before they are incorporated into the IC manual, which should be available in every clinical area in the hospital.

The IC team is responsible for regular updating of the polices in the manual.

Establishing an infection control programme

The IC team is responsible for drawing up infection control policies for consideration by the ICC. This is a slow process and must advance step by step. Some hospital practice is based on past experience, tradition, and policies adopted from other hospitals and radical changes in policy, although necessary, may cause resentment and hostility. The recommended procedure is:

1. Identify interested ward personnel.
2. Identify funding (if any).

3. Study existing practices and assess whether change is required—change should not be made just for the sake of it. Policies based on practices from other hospitals, where the problems may be different, should only be adopted if applicable to the current situation.
4. Formulate simple, easy-to-follow policies.
5. Modify policies accordingly, without compromising the infection control.
6. Use common sense in decision-making.
7. Maintain standards of care.
8. Inform everyone in the hospital of the changes—this can be done via the various representatives on the ICC. The IC team should ensure that information is passed on to any area not covered by the ICC. One means of dispersing information is via the administrator's office to all heads of department.
9. Educate staff—formally and informally.
10. Implement changes gradually.
11. Incorporate written policies in the IC manual.
12. Monitor the IC policies. This should be on-going and has to be carried out with tact and with the co-operation of the hospital staff. It may be incorporated into surveillance and data collection, which is a useful means of communicating with the hospital staff.

Formulating policies

A policy is a consensus decision that outlines the action to be taken in respect of a given situation. It should be simple, easy to follow and fall within the working practices of the hospital—it will be impossible to implement a policy that no-one understands or can follow. For a policy to be effective, it should:

- be formulated only after wide consultation;
- be simple;
- take into account current procedures in the working area;
- take into account any difficulties that may arise during implementation;
- have the co-operation of the staff—it should not be imposed upon them;

- be disseminated widely and followed up regularly;
- take into account suitable alternatives;
- take into account costs and the availability of medical supplies;
- be followed up regularly.

There are two types of policy:

1. *General.* These are overall policies applicable to the whole hospital and are based on general principles of infection control, e.g. disinfectants waste disposal, sharps disposal, etc.
2. *Specific.* These are devised for each unit and cater for the specific requirement of the unit, e.g. burns, oncology, operating theatres, etc.

When setting up a policy:

- A detailed study of the existing practices and the reasons behind them is essential.
- Identify the areas that require change or improvement.
- Draft a policy.
- Identify the departments that will be affected by the change in policy.
- Consult all affected departments about the draft policy via the ICC. Ask for opinions and advice to be given by a certain deadline.
- Consider these points; formulate a definitive policy;
- Make simple and practical (workable) recommendations.

IC policies should be formulated for:

- disinfection;
- antibiotics;
- sterile services;
- waste disposal and handling;
- sharps disposal;
- isolation facilities for patients;
- kitchen and catering;
- planning and development;
- purchasing of new equipment (which might require sterilization and disinfection);
- decontamination of equipment servicing.

Policies may also be needed for specialized areas such as the intensive care unit, operating theatres, the burns unit and the bone marrow transplant unit.

Education

Education and training of all hospital staff is essential to increase awareness of the importance of infection control. All members of staff must understand what is happening and why—this is the essence of a successful IC policy. For example, domestic staff must understand that sweeping disperses dust and environmental bacteria, and should therefore be replaced by damp cleaning. Student nurses and doctors should have training in infection control as part of their education and refresher courses should be available for qualified staff as a continuous and on-going process.

Summary

- The ICC comprises the IC team and representatives from all other interested department and groups.
- The IC comprises the IC doctor, the IC nurse, an administrator, and (sometimes) a medical technician.
- Infection control policy should be:
  —drawn up only after consultation with clinicians and staff;
  —incorporated in the IC manual;
  —monitored by the IC team.

Part 2
The policies

4. *Preventive measures*

Disinfection policy

Disinfection and sterilization are necessary to prevent cross-infection from equipment, surfaces and skin and are used in all hospitals:

- **Decontamination** renders an article safe for handling.

- **Disinfection** is used to reduce the number of micro-organisms on an object or surface, although the disinfectants used rarely destroy all the micro-organisms they come into contact with.

- **Sterilization** (absolute term) is used to remove all living micro-organisms from an object by one of two methods:
  —*Heat sterilization.* This is the cheapest, safest, and most effective method of sterilization.
  —*Cold sterilization.* The only reliable method of cold sterilization is prolonged exposure to 2 per cent glutaraldehyde, although this can become inactivated under adverse conditions. Cold sterilization should only be used on heat-sensitive items of equipment (e.g. endoscopes) and must be used with caution and within the COSHH regulations (see Health and Safety, p. 172).

Many hospitals have no clear disinfection policy and practices are often based more on tradition and habit than on logic. However, a sensible disinfection policy can save the hospital money and reduce the number of nosocomial and cross-infections.

Principles of sterilization and disinfection

Sterilization

Sterilization should be used on all heat-stable equipment where possible, and most clinical equipment requires disinfection and heat sterilization. The exceptions are heat-sensitive items, which should be sterilized with prolonged exposure to 2 per cent glutaraldehyde (see above).

Disinfection

Disinfectants:

- Are most efficient if used according to instruction and at the correct (optimum) dilution.
- Differ in their properties depending on the circumstances.
- May be rapidly inactivated by organic matter. Any object that is to be disinfected must therefore be cleaned thoroughly with warm water and detergent prior to disinfection.

Sustained-action disinfectants should be used for hand hygiene by staff (see Hand Disinfection, p. 44) and to cleanse patients' skin and mucous membranes. Alcohol preparations over 40 per cent are no longer recommended for operations because of the risk of fire when used in conjunction with diathermy (see p. 141).

Hard Surfaces

Hard surfaces do not require disinfectants—warm water with detergent is usually sufficient to remove all organic contamination. The exceptions are where persistence of potentially dangerous pathogens, such as hepatitis B or HIV, is suspected, when the surface should be wiped with disinfectant (see p. 95).

Equipment

See page 120.

Rules for the use of disinfectants

- Follow the manufacturers' instructions.
- Check the expiry date of the solution.
- Ensure that the optimum dilution is used.
- Always wash and clean articles before disinfection.
- **DO NOT REFILL DISINFECTANT CONTAINERS** without sterilizing the container between each use—topping up is **NOT** allowed.
- Disinfectants should be supplied ready for use from the pharmacy.
- Empty containers should be returned to the pharmacy. New

stocks should be supplied on receipt of the empty containers. DO NOT DISCARD EMPTY CONTAINERS OR USE THEM TO STORE ANY OTHER SOLUTIONS—this is dangerous and must be discouraged. Chemicals can be harmful when used in the wrong situation.

• Disinfectants should not be used to sterilize instruments or equipment (unless specified in the disinfectant policy, e.g. endoscopes).

• Open containers of disinfectant should not be tolerated in any hospital environment as there is a serious risk of contamination with multiply antibiotic-resistant bacteria, such as *Pseudomonas* species and spores.

• Where disinfectants are indicated for use on surfaces WIPE—DO NOT BATHE. Bathing wastes disinfectant.

Drawing up a disinfection policy

• List the purposes for which disinfectants are currently used.

• Eliminate disinfectants where:
  —heat sterilization is required;
  —more reliable means are available;
  —no disinfection is necessary;
  —it is not cost effective, e.g. for disposable, single-use items.

• Select an effective disinfectant for the remaining indications.

• Arrange for disinfectants to be distributed to the points of use—wards, departments, etc.—at the optimum dilution.

• Ensure that no further dilution occurs at the points of use.

• Return the containers to the pharmacy after use.

• Ensure that expiry dates are adhered to.

Table 4.1 gives an example of a disinfection policy.

The role of the pharmacy

The pharmacy should ensure that:

• The disinfectant containers are thoroughly cleaned, washed, and dried.

Table 4.1 Example of a disinfection policy]

Area to be disinfected	Disinfectant
Skin	
injection site	70 % isopropyl alcohol
antiseptic hand wash	Aqueous 4 % chlorhexidine
staff hand disinfection between patients in high risk areas	0.5 % (w/v) + 70% isopropyl alcohol (Hibisol)
Routine preoperative skin	Chlorhexidine or povidone iodine
Surfaces	
ward floors	Warm water and detergent
operating theatre	Warm water and detergent. Dry Spot cleaning for blood and body fluid as below
Equipment	
endoscopes and other fibre optics	2% glutaraldehyde for 10 min (immerse for 3 h for tuberculosis)
Body fluids	
laboratory use	Hypochlorite diluted 1 in 10 (available chlorine 10,000 p.p.m.)
spillage of blood/body fluids in wards/clinical areas	Hypochlorite 1 in 100 (available chlorine 100 p.p.m.)

- The containers are filled with the correct solution, at the right dilution.
- The containers are clearly labelled with:
  —contents;
  —in-use dilution;
  —expiry date.
- None of the disinfectants are exposed to inactivating substances, such as cork, rubber, or incompatible detergents.
- The disinfectants are diluted by a knowledgeable person, in manageable quantities, e.g. 500 ml or less. This will reduce waste and the chance that partially filled bottles will be left on the ward.

Reasons for inactivation of disinfectants
The reasons of ineffective disinfection are shown in Table 4.2.

Table 4.2 The reasons for inactivation of disinfectants

Reason	Remedy
Inaccurate dilution	Ensure clear instructions
	Make up in the pharmacy
	DO NOT TOP UP
Contaminated water for dilution	Use distilled or deionized water
Incompatible containers	Check compatibility
	Avoid plastic and rubber
Unsuitable closures	Do not use cork stoppers or caps
Unfavourable pH	Check pH compatibility with cation and anion detergents
	Check mixing with other detergents, e.g. quaternary ammonium compounds
Use with unsuitable materials	Do not use with rayon, cotton wool or gauze

Summary

- Sterilize all non-heat-sensitive equipment.
- Disinfect heat-sensitive equipment.
- Use disinfectants properly (see p. 30).
- Design and implement a disinfectant policy (see p. 30).

Waste disposal

Hospitals generate enormous amounts of waste. In 1991 an estimated 100 000 tonnes of waste was generated in British NHS hospitals (Department of Health Press Release H91/616). This amounted to, on average, between 0.5 and 0.6 kg of waste per bed per day. Effective disposal of this large quantity of waste is best done by dividing the waste into categories and using different methods of disposal for the various categories.

Unfortunately, hospitals in countries with inadequate disposal facilities may dump contaminated hospital waste on open rubbish tips. This presents a great risk to the people, especially children, who scavenge in these rubbish piles, which are also breeding grounds for pests and vermin, and which contribute to the spread

Table 4.3 The properties of disinfectants

Property	Disinfectant						
	Glutar-aldehyde	Hypo-chlorite	Phenolic	Alcohol	Chlorhex-idine	Povidone iodine	Quaternary ammonium compounds
Antimicrobial activity							
vegetative bacteria	+	+	+	+	+	+	+
mycobacteria	+	+	+	+	−	−	−
viruses	+	+	+	+	−	+	+/−
spores	+	+	−	−	−	+	−
Effects							
inactivation[1]	Yes	No	No	No	No	No	Yes
corrosive/damaging[2]	No	Yes	Yes	No	No	No	No
toxic/irritant[3]	Yes	Yes	Yes	No	No	No	No

[1] Inactivation of disinfectant in the presence of organic matter.
[2] To equipment.
[3] To staff/patients.

of disease. All hospital waste should be disposed of so that is presents no risk of injury/contamination.

Types of hospital waste

Clinical waste

Clinical waste is generated during routine patient care, surgery and in high risk units. It is potentially dangerous and presents a high risk of infection to the general population and to the hospital staff. It should be clearly labelled **HIGH RISK**.

Examples of clinical waste include:

- soiled dressings;
- body fluids;
- amputated limbs;
- i.v. needles and syringes;
- drainage bags;
- pathology waste;
- blood products.

Laboratory waste

This also comes under the **HIGH RISK** category and should be autoclaved before leaving the department. It should be clearly labelled **BIOHAZARD**.

Non-clinical waste

This includes wrapping paper, office paper, and plastic that has not been in contact with patient body fluids. Although it is of no potential harm it is bulky and is therefore difficult to dispose of.

Kitchen waste

This includes swill, left-over food, and dirty water. It is a potential source of pests and vermin, such as cockroaches, mice, and rats and is thus an indirect potential hazard to the staff and patients in a hospital.

Radioactive waste

This is not an infection control issue and will not be considered here. However, provisions must be made for safe disposal of radioactive waste.

Colour-coding

A simple colour-coding system should be used to separate waste so that the different components can be treated safely. The UK has a national colour-coding system, which demarcates different types of waste and soiled and infected laundry. The colour-coding is consistent between hospitals and is designed to be used easily by all staff (Table 4.4).

Table 4.4 An example of a colour-coding system for hospital waste

Type of waste	Colour
Wards/department	
clinical	Yellow
non-clinical	Black
Hospital laundry	
soiled/infected	Red
dirty/used	White
theatre	Green/blue
Kitchen	Different coloured gloves used for cooking and cleaning equipment

To ensure the smooth operation of a colour-coding policy different coloured containers should be provided throughout the hospital so that the waste can be separated at source:

- Wards should be provided with two separate colour-coded containers—one for *clinical* and one for *non-clinical waste*.
- All waste from operating theatres should be defined as *clinical waste*.
- Office waste is usually paper and is defined as *non-clinical waste*.
- All waste leaving the pathology department should be defined as *clinical waste* and must be rendered safe before disposal. All

pathology waste in the UK, especially from bacteriology and virology, is autoclaved prior to incineration.

- A separate colour should be used in each kitchen work area (see p. 154).

Points to be considered when formulating a colour-coding policy

Separation of waste

- Waste should be separated at source.
- All high risk waste should be clearly labelled.
- Colour-coded plastic bags (minimum gauge 225 μm for high risk waste and 100 μm for low risk waste) should be used. The destination of the bags will depend on the colour coding (see Disposal of Waste, p. 38).

Plastic may be considered an unnecessary expense in some countries and it may be cheaper to use thick, leak-proof paper bags (these are often manufactured locally and are therefore readily available). These paper bags can be labelled with colour-coded strips and should be placed in colour-coded metal bins in the wards and departments and are an equally effective means of separating waste at its source.

A separate bin should be provided in the kitchen or sluice for the disposal of food waste in those countries where the patients' visitors and relatives act as attendants. These bins should be emptied at least once daily and the internal lining should be replaced after each emptying.

Storage of waste

- The colour-coded bags in the wards should be emptied when they are two-thirds full. They should be tied securely at the neck and labelled clearly.
- The bags should be carried by the neck (so that they swing away from the body) and taken to a predesignated area for collection.
- The collection staff should ensure that the waste is segregated properly according to the colour-coding and sent to the appropriate destination.
- The bags should be stored in vermin-and vandal-proof cages ready for transportation to their destination.

Handling waste

- The colour-coded bags should be handled only after they have been secured.
- The bags should be carried by the neck.
- Porters should wear protective clothing, e.g. heavy-duty gauntlets or gloves and overalls, when transporting the bags.
- If external contamination occurs, the soiled bag should be placed inside a clean, new bag (double bagging), which should be tied securely.
- Porters are perfectly within their rights to refuse to remove the waste if sharps or items liable to cause injury are found in the wrong bag.

UNDER NO CIRCUMSTANCES SHOULD ANY MEMBER OF STAFF PUT THEIR HANDS INTO ANY WASTE CONTAINER.

Transportation of waste

- *Collection.* The bags are collected by a porter with a dedicated van or cage trolley, who separates them according to their colour-coding.
- *Transportation:*
  —non-clinical waste is taken to a compactor and clinical waste to the incinerator;
  —the external transport system, whether provided by the local authority or by a private contractor, should be by dedicated vans.
- *Loading.* Both the compactor and the incinerator should be loaded automatically where possible.
- *Cleaning.* All vehicles used to carry waste must be emptied and washed down daily. Bleach should be used if a leakage has occurred.

Disposal of waste

- *Non-clinical waste.* After compaction, this can be disposed of at a land-fill site. In the UK, this is usually organized by the local authority or by a private contractor.
- *Clinical waste.* This requires incineration or, failing this, must be covered with lime and buried (see Liming, below).

● *Kitchen waste.* This must be used or destroyed on the day of preparation. Most kitchens have a waste disposal macerator but, in developing countries, the food may be distributed to the needy. The policy of selling the food as swill to farmers is no longer recommended (see Kitchens, p. 157).

Incineration facilities In the UK, these are either on site or at a central area provided by the local authority.

A large hospital may find it cost-effective to invest in an incinerator. Small or medium-sized incinerators, burning at 1300–1500°C or higher, are now available and it is possible to recycle up to 60 per cent of the heat produced by these incinerators into energy for the hospital. Income generation—selling incinerator time to other hospitals—is also possible. This will eleviate their problems of waste disposal and the incinerator may become self-financing.

A good modern incinerator which fulfils the new legal requirements is an advantage, particularly if facilities for land-fill are not available, as it enables the safe disposal of all non-clinical and clinical waste, including sharps and expired pharmacy products.

Liming Where incineration facilities are not available, clinical waste can be treated with lime and buried in the hospital grounds. To do this safely:

1. Dig a pit, approximately 2.5 m deep.
2. Spread a layer of up to 75 cm of clinical waste across the bottom of the pit.
3. Add a layer of lime.
4. Continue layering every 75 cm until the pit is filled to within 0.5 m of the ground.
5. Fill the pit with earth before starting another.

Liming is the cheapest and most effective means of getting rid of clinical waste in areas where incineration facilities are not available. Care should be taken not to bury non-biodegradable products, e.g. plastic bags. Tins containing sharps should be buried. Use paper bags when liming.

Non-clinical waste This should not be treated with lime but should be removed by the local authority or an independent contractor and disposed of independently or at the municipal dump. NO CLINICAL WASTE, NEEDLES OR SYRINGES SHOULD BE SENT TO THE MUNICIPAL DUMP—THE HOSPITAL MUST

NOT BE RESPONSIBLE FOR INCREASING THE RISK OF DISEASE.

Protection and training of staff

- All staff handling clinical waste must be adequately trained and aware of the protocol for action in the event of accidental inoculation or body contamination.
- All staff must be provided with adequate protective clothing and replacement garments.
- Hepatitis B immunization should be offered to all staff and proper records of such immunization should kept by the Occupational Health Department.

Sharps

There is a very real risk of acquiring blood-borne diseases from sharps contaminated with blood products. All sharps, including **FINE-BORE** needles, must be single-use only:

- Needles and syringes should *never* be recycled, no matter what the circumstances.
- Needles should *never* be reused for injecting drugs into an i.v. giving system.

Needles *must* be sterile and this cannot be guaranteed if they are recycled, even if they are autoclaved.

The financial savings made by recycling sharps do not justify the risks involved: it has been estimated that 17 per cent of sharps injuries occur before or during use, 70 per cent occur after use but before disposal and that 13 per cent occur after disposal. Approximately 40 per cent of these accidents are avoidable, and most of these are resheathing incidents.

Broken glass

Broken glass should be included in the sharps category. To dispose safely with broken glass:

1. Wear thick gloves.
2. Use newspaper or similar thick paper to collect the glass.

3. Wrap the glass securely in the paper.
4. Put the wrapped glass in a cardboard box, which should be marked **BROKEN GLASS—HANDLE WITH CARE** or with yellow **BIOHAZARD** tape.
5. Tell the porters that the box contains broken glass.

Sharps containers

In the UK these must comply with BS 89/52770 (May 1990). All sharps containers must:

- Be leak-proof and puncture-proof.
- Have a handle that allows lifting with only one hand (so that the container falls away from the body when it is carried).
- Have a non-reopenable lid.
- Be designed to be used with one hand.
- Carry a **BIOLOGICAL HAZARD** sign.
- Be sealed and replaced when it is no more than two-thirds full.

Different sized sharps containers should always be available.

Disposal

Sharps containers are clinical waste and should be put into clinical waste bags before being incinerated.

Ideally, all sharps containers should be incinerated but, if this is not possible, they should be buried in impervious tin containers and limed with the other clinical waste (see p. 39). Whichever method is used, there must be no possibility of injury from the sharps.

Accidents

Staff safety is very important and inoculation accidents must be avoided. Where such an accident occurs, it must be documented by the senior manager and reported to the Occupational Health Department and the Infection Control Team immediately so that appropriate action can be taken (see Hepatitis Policy, p. 174). In the UK, all injuries must be recorded in an accident book in accordance with the Social Security Act (1975).

There must be a clearly defined policy on the action to be taken when a sharps injury occurs and all staff should be aware of this policy. Immunization should have been made available to all staff considered to be at risk of a sharps injury and counselling facilities must be available after any accident (see Blood-borne Diseases, p. 97 and Occupational Health, p. 107).

Summary

- Colour-code the different types of hospital waste (see p. 36).
- Dispose of the different types of waste correctly:
  —*Clinical waste* should be incinerated (or buried with lime; see p. 39).
  —*Non-clinical waste* should be compacted and sent to a land-fill site (or incinerated; see p. 39).
  —*Needles and sharps* are clinical waste and should be incinerated (or buried in impervious containers with lime; see p. 59).
  —*Broken glass* is clinical waste and should be incinerated (or buried with lime; see p. 59).
  —*Kitchen waste* should be disposed of via waste disposal unit or safely by a local arrangement (see p. 157).
- Never recycle used needles or syringes.
- Dispose of all sharps in a clearly labelled sharps container (see p. 41).

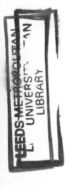

Aseptic procedure

Aseptic procedure is the introduction of a sterile item such as an i.v. cannula or urinary catheter into a patient using a no-touch technique. During the procedure:

- the entry site must be properly cleaned;
- the hands of the staff must be disinfected (and gloved);
- sterility of the article is maintained by minimizing contact with non-sterile surfaces.

Hands are the most common source of cross-infection. A clear policy on hand disinfection is therefore essential and should be followed meticulously by all members of staff and by patients' relatives. In countries with a shortage of water, or where the quality of water is substandard, methods of disinfection other than using soap and water should be considered. The use of gloves, for example, reduces the transmission of bacteria, although hand disinfection is still recommended after the gloves have been taken off, to remove any contamination that might have occurred via small punctures.

Hand washing

There two types of hand washing:

1. *Social hand washing*. This should be carried out:
   —routinely before and after coming into contact with patients;
   —when starting work;
   —when going off-duty;
   —when they become visibly dirty;
   —when they are contaminated with body fluids or organic matter;
   —after visiting the toilet;
   —after removing gloves;
   —after a non-sterile procedure;
   —contact with patients during ward rounds or routine procedures such as bed-making or lifting should be followed by decontamination of the hands with alcohol chlorhexidine or a soap and water hand-wash.
2. *Aseptic hand-washing*. This type of hand washing should be used when as aseptic procedure is about to be performed on a patient (e.g. introducing central venous pressure lines, peripheral cannulae or urinary catheters). It is a shorter version of the surgical hand wash (see Operating Theatres, p. 142) and requires meticulous cleaning of the hands and the use of a sustained action disinfectant. It is usually accompanied by the wearing of gloves.

Procedure for hand-washing

- Remove all rings, jewellery (including watch) and roll up the sleeves.
- Wet the hands under running water and apply a recommended amount of the hand-wash provided to the palms of the hands.
- Rub to make a lather.

- Rub the hands together and then cup them around each other to massage all the finger tips properly, massaging the thumbs and the webs of the fingers.
- Wash the wrists and backs of the hands.
- Rinse the hands thoroughly under running water.
- Dry thoroughly with several pieces of paper towel or single-use cotton towels.

If washing for an aseptic procedure:

- Do not touch any non-sterile surface.
- Wear gloves.
- Remove gloves after the procedure, wash hands and dry thoroughly.

Hand disinfection

Sustained-action disinfectants with alcohol (rub) should be used:

- when moving from one patient to another;
- after non-sterile duties not involving body fluids;
- after handling or touching a potentially contaminated surface;
- before touching a neutropenic or high-dependence patient.

All hand disinfection agents should be kept in a sterile dispenser that delivers a known quantity of soap or disinfectant. The container and nozzle must be cleaned regularly to prevent contamination and blocking. Open containers of disinfectant and soap should not be left on ward wash-hand basins as they can become contaminated with bacteria. When empty, the disinfectant containers should be returned to the Pharmacy or Domestic Department to be washed, cleaned and refilled. Defective pumps must be replaced immediately.

Soap and water

Soap and water remove most organic contamination and are acceptable as a social-hand wash (see p. 43). However, bars of soap may be left lying in pools of water, where they become contaminated with multiply antibiotic-resistant Gram-negative bacilli, which are then transferred to the hands of staff and then to patients. If bar soaps are used they should be stored dry—either on a piece of string or fixed to the wall by magnet holders. Medicated soap, which incorporates a bactericidal agent (e.g. Triclosan or Irgasan—Cidal soap) is useful in reducing the transmission of methicillin-resistant *Staphylococcus aureus*. Soap and water should be supplemented with an alcohol-containing sustained action disinfectant prior to carrying out an aseptic technique.

Sustained-action disinfectants

Sustained-action disinfectants (e.g. chlorhexidine and povidone iodine) remove organic contamination and, with repeated use, maintain low bacterial hand-counts. They are recommended prior to an aseptic technique. There is a reported level of allergy to these disinfectants, although the most common reason for 'allergy' is inadequate drying of the hands. Hand-creams may be applied after washing and drying the hands.

Some users are genuinely allergic to chlorhexidine and alternatives (e.g. povidone iodine) may be used.

Alcohol-based sustained-action disinfectants

Alcohol-based sustained-action disinfectants (e.g. Hibisol) are extremely useful and are an excellent means of providing hand disinfection in areas where washing facilities are lacking or where the staff are too busy to disinfect their hands between patients. A container of alcohol-based disinfectant beside each bed in a high dependency unit results in a significant increase in compliance with disinfection policy. A container placed on the clinical notes trolley is useful for hand disinfection between patients during ward rounds.

Alcohol-based disinfectants are also useful in countries where hand-washing facilities are lacking and in remote regions when minor surgical procedures are performed outside the operating theatre. Alcohol (70%) alone is cheaper and as effective as 'Hibisol'.

70 per cent isopropyl alcohol

This may be the only disinfectant available in countries that cannot afford sustained-action disinfectants. It is sold world-wide as 'rubbing alcohol' for sprains and aches. Its disadvantage is that it causes dryness of the skin and allergic rashes. As well as being used to disinfect the hands, it may also be applied to gloves to reduce bacterial counts and so allow the safe re-use of gloves in non-sterile procedures.

Hand-wash basins

These should be available in all wards, treatment rooms, sluice rooms and isolation cubicles. A clinical hand-wash basin has:

- elbow-operated mixer taps;
- a deep bowl to avoid splashing and contamination;
- no overflow;
- no recesses where water may collect;
- no drain-hole plug, so that water cannot be held in the basin.

Hand operated single taps should be turned off with the paper-or cloth towel that was used to dry the hands.

Wash-hand basins should be used for hand-washing only and should have a clearly displayed sign: **CAUTION—HOT WATER** and **HAND-WASH ONLY.**

The two-bowl system with a communal towel is not recommended—it is a source of cross-infection.

Siting the wash basins

- Wash basins should be in the easy sight and reach of all hospital staff and visitors (no-one will use a wash basin they cannot see).
- Basins should have adequate, wall-mounted hand disinfectants.
- Drying facilities should be close by.

In some countries, the wash-hand basin on the ward is used as a kitchen sink by the patients' relatives. This has disadvantages:

- the staff cannot use the wash basin for hand disinfection;
- the sink may be blocked with food debris and over-flow;
- vermin and pests may be attracted to the ward;
- it is extremely unsightly.

Bins *must* be provided to dispose of waste for relatives and visitors use in the kitchen, or sluice, and relatives should be educated about hand hygiene.

Hand drying

Drying is an essential part of hand disinfection. Wet hands have higher bacterial counts and permanently wet hands become chapped and dry.

Paper towels

These are most often used to dry the hands. However, the quality is usually poor and several sheets are needed to the dry the hands properly. A good absorbent quality is recommended.

Cotton towels

These are perfectly acceptable for social hand-washing provided that they are on a roller and are laundered regularly. A small face-towel for single use (i.e. is laundered before re-use) is also acceptable. Common-use cotton towels that are left lying next to a sink are dangerous and can result in cross-infection with Gram-positive cocci and Gram-negative bacilli.

Air hand-dryers

These are becoming popular in some countries. However, they should not be installed inside high dependency areas with susceptible patients, because there is a risk of bacterial dispersal from aerosols. The drier should be mounted on a wall near the wash-basin, but away from a clinical area. Hot and cold air dryers are equally effective. Alternative means of hand drying should be considered.

Intravenous therapy

At any given time, 25 per cent of in-patients will have a peripheral cannula *in situ*. This is one of the most common invasive procedures performed in hospital and yet it is also one of the most neglected in terms of hospital-acquired infection (see also Sharps Disposal Policy, p. 40 and Disposable Equipment, p. 124).

Possible sources of infection

- Factors related to equipment and fluids:
  —Cannula material that is itself thrombogenic. For example, polyethylene and polypropylene are more reactive than Teflon,

which is in turn more reactive than steel or silicone-coated Teflon.
—Contaminated administration sets.
—Hypodermic needles used as air inlets.
—Three-way taps and stop cocks.
—Infusion fluids.
—Dirty dressings, adhesive tapes, or film.
—Contaminated splints used to stabilize joints.
—Large bandages used to cover the insertion site (these can be contaminated by the patient's blood and body fluids).

- Factors relating to insertion and duration:
  —Patient's skin flora if skin disinfection is inadequate.
  —Hands of staff, other patients or visitors.
  —Contaminated disinfectants.
  —Unstable cannulae—movement increases the risk of bacterial contamination.
  —Cannulae left in for over 72 hours.
  —Insertion of cannula into a previously infected vein. Alternate arms should be used for i.v. therapy that lasts longer than 72 hours.
  —Septicaemia (endogenous infection).

Procedure for inserting i.v. cannulae

1. Ensure that the patient is comfortable and aware of the procedure—this reduces anxiety.
2. Collect all equipment necessary to set up an i.v. infusion.
3. Apply a tourniquet to the patient's non-dominant forearm.
4. Disinfect the i.v. insertion site with 70 per cent isopropyl alcohol for at least 30 seconds and allow to dry before inserting the cannula. (NOTE: the i.v. site should not be touched after disinfection. If the tourniquet has been in place for a sufficient length of time touching should not be necessary.)
5. Disinfect hands.
6. Select a cannula that will fit easily into the vein—size 18 or 20 gauge is usually appropriate. The correct sized cannula reduces trauma and congestion of the vein.
7. Insert the cannula as swiftly and as aseptically as possible. Do not attempt repeated insertions with the same cannula. If the

first insertion is not successful the procedure should be repeated with a new cannula.

8. Look out for flash-back and then advance the cannula slowly.
9. Anchor the cannula with clean tape, using a U-technique:
   —Place a piece of adhesive tape between the hub of the cannula and the patient's arm—the adhesive surface should face upwards.
   —Attach the tape to the undersurface of the hub of the cannula.
   —Fold the tape at right angles on itself so that the adhesive surface faces down and is parallel with the cannula shaft (forming pseudo wings for a straight-hubbed cannula and adhering to the flaps of a winged cannula).
   —Lay another piece of tape across the hub, adhesive surface down, to hold the hub in place on the patient's arm. Loop and hold the administration tube under this piece of tape.
   —Lay another piece of tape across the U-arms of the tape and fix firmly. This leaves the cannula firmly anchored and the site of insertion free for inspection.
10. Release the tourniquet.
11. Connect up the administration set.
12. Clean the site with a 70 per cent isopropyl alcohol swab.
13. Leave the site visible and dry.
14. Discard all sharps carefully in the container provided (see Sharps Disposal, p. 40).
15. Wash and dry hands.

Maintenance of i.v. lines

- Inspect regularly for swelling, or signs of infection.
- Keep site clean and dry.
- Consider resiting the cannula after 72 hours.
- Change administration sets within 72 hours (Note: a change in solution may require a change of administration set).
- Wipe the hub of the cannula with an alcohol-impregnated swab before attaching the administration set. The Luer lock should be kept as clean and dry as possible.

Central venous pressure (CVP) lines

The insertion of CVP lines is an aseptic procedure and should be carried out in sterile drapes, gown and gloves. Masks are not necessary. A suggested procedure is:

1. Place the patient in the Trendleberg position.
2. Surround the site with sterile drapes and clean thoroughly with a sustained-action disinfectant. Allow site to dry.
3. Insert the central line with minimum trauma.
4. Leave the site clean and dry after insertion.
5. Spray the site with povidone iodine (if this is hospital policy).
6. Cover the site with a sterile (transparent) dressing for easy inspection. Sterile gauze may be used but should not be covered with an impervious dressing, as this increases the risk of infection.
7. Clean the hub with an alcohol swab before each connection to the administration set.
8. Check drug incompatibilities with the pharmacist.
9. Non-tunnelled central lines should be changed after 5 days.
10. Tunnelled central lines should be removed if infected or at the end of therapy.

Fluids and hyperalimentation should be administered via a *closed system*. Potential points of entry for bacteria occur when the system is broken, e.g. by three-way taps and stop corks. Suitable alternatives, e.g. multi-flo systems, can be shut off independently and the administration set changed as required. Triple-lumen catheters can also be connected and disconnected individually.

Discontinued administration sets should not be left hanging on the drip stand awaiting re-connection.

I.v. devices cannot be sterilized with antibiotics and must be removed if the patient becomes pyrexial.

Bacteriology investigation as part of after-care of i.v. lines

Patients with i.v. devices can become pyrexial. All such cases require bacteriological investigation:

- The insertion site should be inspected for redness or swelling—if it appears infected, the intravenous device should be removed and sent (in a sterile container) for bacteriological examination.
- A wound swab should be taken from the site of insertion.
- A blood culture should be taken from a peripheral site, preferably the opposite arm.

- A blood culture should be taken from the central line.
- *Chemotherapy.* A patient showing signs of infection during a course of chemotherapy, when the central line cannot be removed, should be given appropriate antibiotics (e.g. a glycopeptide alone or with an aminoglycoside) until the end of therapy. The line should then be removed and sent for culture.
- *Hyperalimentation.* There seems to be no advantage in covering the feeding period with antibiotics and it is best to replace the line as soon as possible, under antibiotic cover (to reduce the risk of septicaemia), and then maintain therapy for 5–7 days if clinically indicated.
- The after-care of i.v. catheters is crucial. The site should be inspected daily and dressed aseptically when any moisture around the insertion site is noted.

Urinary catheterization

Urinary catheterization is an aseptic procedure but is a common cause of bacteraemia, which can occur during insertion or removal of the catheter. Repeated catheterization causes trauma and results in infection. Patients should catheterized only if clinically indicated, and certainly not for the convenience of the nursing staff.

Suggested catheterization procedure

1. Inform the patient of the reasons for catheterization and explain the procedure.
2. Lay all necessary equipment on a trolley.
3. Wash and dry hands thoroughly (see p. 44).
4. Select a catheter that fits the urethra without traumatizing the patient.
5. If the patient is male, draw back the foreskin and clean the glans thoroughly with sterile water to remove secretions. Disinfectants are not required.
6. Insert the nozzle of the tube of anaesthetic jelly being used (e.g. lignocaine) and squeeze 2–3 ml of sterile jelly into the urethra. Multiple-use tubes are not recommended because they can become contaminated and increase cross-infection.
7. Leave the anaesthetic to take effect (2–3 minutes)

8. Insert the catheter gently—advance it by holding the inner sterile sleeve.
9. Collect the urine in a suitable container.
10. Fill the balloon with 5–10 ml sterile water.
11. Anchor the catheter to the patient's thigh.
12. Connect up the urine drainage bag and hang it below the level of the bed to stop reflux.
13. Wash and dry hands.

It is important to use the correct urinary catheter for the condition (Tables 4.5 and 4.6). Foley's catheters require no more than 5–10 ml water, while haemostasis catheters require 30 ml. The balloon can cause obstruction and stasis of the urine if it is too large, thus increasing the risk of infection.

Table 4.5 Types of urinary catheter and indications (as used at the North Middlesex Hospital)

Use	Type of catheter	Material	Size
Residual urine; intermittent self-catheterization	Nelaton	Plastic	One size
Short-term (up to 3 weeks)	Foley two-way	Latex/Teflon-coated	
Irrigation (closed system)	Foley three-way	Latex/Teflon-coated	
Long-term (up to 3 months)	Biocath	Hydrogel-coated	
Haematuria	Folatex	Latex/Teflon-coated	22 and 24 gauge

Table 4.6 General specifications for all catheters

Indication	Size	
Retention--general	Balloon	5–10 ml
Haematuria		30 ml
Children	Charriére	6–10 Foley gauge
Adults	Charriére	12–16 Foley gauge
Urology only	Charriére	18+ Foley gauge
Males	Standard length of catheter 30 cm	
Females	Short catheter (female)	

Emptying the drainage bag

This should be done wearing non-sterile gloves and via the drainage tap at the bottom of the bag. if the bag does not have a tap, replace it when full. DO NOT DISCONNECT THE BAG TO EMPTY AND THEN RECONNECT IT. If, for financial reasons, drainage systems have to be recycled, heat disinfection cannot be considered and re-use is not generally recommended.

With proper handling, drainage bags with taps can be left in situ for long periods and are mor cost-effective in the long run.

Long-term catheters

Several long-term urinary catheters are available (Table 4.5). The choice of catheter is important because frequent changing is not advisable due to the increased risk of bacteraemia. In the UK continence nurse advisors are available to give advice on the selection of long-term catheters.

The care of long-term catheters is usually managed by the patients if they are at home and by the nurses if in hospital.

Intermittent catheterization

Self-catheterization is recommended for patients with chronic urinary stasis. Most patients can be taught to catheterize themselves intermittently and the risk of infection is not increased. Disposable intermittent catheters are recommended because re-usable metal or rubber catheters must be properly sterilized and, although the risk of infection is not increased (because the patient is recycling to him-/herself) the irritation from the chemicals used for disinfection can be a problem.

Recycling of urinary catheters

See page 51.

Wound inspection and care

Surgical wounds

These should be sterile at operation and in most cases, after operation. Infection can be introduced during the operation or postoperatively via hands and contaminated dressings. It is best not interfere with surgical wounds unless indicated, e.g. if there are signs of infection and a change of dressing is required.

Traumatic wounds

These are potentially contaminated with environmental and faecal bacteria and may become colonized with hospital pathogens, which may then be transferred to other patients via the hands of the staff.

Suggested procedure for wound care

Wounds must not be touched with dirty hands and wound care should be an aseptic procedure:

1. Lay up a trolley with a sterile wound dressing pack.
2. Remove old dressing and inspect the wound.
3. Wash and dry hands.
4. Clean wound thoroughly, using forceps and cotton wool or gauze soaked in a cleaning solution. Do not use hands.
5. Exude any fluids from an infected wound by pressing with two sterile gauze pieces held with two forceps.
6. Take specimens of pus or exudate for bacteriological examination.
7. Apply necessary medication.
8. Wipe the wound site as dry as possible.
9. Cover the wound if indicated.
10. Discard all dirty dressings in a clinical waste bag.
11. Wash and dry hands.

Individual sterile wound dressing packs containing all the sterile items required to dress a wound should be available from the Sterile Supplies Department. Tightly closed containers of antiseptics (if required) should be stored separately and poured into the sterile gallipot found in the dressing pack; discard what is left over in the gallipot. It is best to buy individual sachets or bottles containing the amount of fluid required for one dressing, if possible.

Although individual sterile wound dressing packs are preferable, many countries still use dressing trolleys, which are left on the ward and are covered with bottles, dressings, and equipment. Potential sources of contamination from these trolleys include:

- Topping-up jars of cotton wool with contaminated disinfectants.

- Putting dirty hands or cheatle forceps into the disinfectant containers (to remove articles) and thereby contaminating the disinfectant.
- Constant use of jars, which are therefore rarely cleaned.
- Contaminated dressings.
- Inactivation of some disinfectants by cotton wool, rayon, and other materials.
- Potential common-source outbreak as a result of spraying the surface of the trolley with contaminated disinfectants.
- Cross-contamination fro the dirty dressing bucket to clean dressings.
- Contamination of common-use equipment (e.g. stethoscope, sphygmomanometer, patella hammer) that is stored on the trolley.
- Lack of hand decontamination facilities between patients.
- Inadequate and infrequent cleaning of the trolley.

Summary

- Hand washing. There are two types:
  —social;
  —aseptic.
- Hand disinfection uses:
  —soap and water;
  —sustained-action disinfectants;
  —alcohol-based disinfectants;
  —70 per cent isopropyl alcohol.
- I.v. therapy. Possible causes of infection are:
  —equipment and fluids;
  —when cannula is inserted;
  —duration of therapy.
- Urinary catheterization:
  —always use correct size catheter;
  —follow recommended insertion procedure (see p. 51);
  —empty or replace drainage bag as appropriate (see p. 53)
- Wounds:
  —follow recommended procedure (see p. 54)
  —avoid using a dressings trolley, if possible (see p. 54).

Sterile services and recycling

The sterile services department

A Sterile Services Department (SSD) is vital for an effective IC programme. Using its expertise and knowledge of sterilization and disinfection to ensure high standards of cleanliness, an SSD always results in long-term savings.

Most hospitals in developed countries have an SSD to deal with hospital and community services and a Theatre Sterile Services Unit (TSSU) to deal with the operating theatres and associated departments. Hospitals in developing countries do not often have the funds to run duplicate units and have a single department, covering all areas. This is perfectly acceptable if the service is satisfactory.

Establishing an SSD

Dirty, recyclable equipment should be collected from the wards and transferred to the SSD, where it is washed, inspected, sterilized, packed, and dispatched back to the wards.

The sterile procedure should be:

- In the ward:
  —Collect instruments that are to be re-used in a clearly labelled container.
  —Arrange for dirty instruments to be delivered to the SSD—DO NOT ATTEMPT TO WASH THEM ON THE WARD.
  —Discard cotton wool balls and dressings for incineration (clinical waste; see p. 38).

- In the SSD:
  —Receive instruments in the dirty area.
  —Wash all equipment in hot water and detergent either mechanically ('no-touch' technique) or manually (use heavy-duty gloves, plastic aprons, and eye protection).
  —Inspect all equipment for cleanliness and damage.
  —Send damaged instruments for repair, or discard.
  —Pack cleaned instruments on trays for ward use.
  —Autoclave trays at recommended temperature and/or disinfect as required.
  —Ensure that the packaged trays are dry—inspect tapes.

—Sort the packaged trays for ward collection.
—Return to the ward clean treatment room.

The layout of the SSD

Ideally, dirty and clean areas should be separated by physical barriers. However, if this is not possible (perhaps because of shortage of space or funds) the same room can be used, provided that:

- the air moves from the clean area to the dirty area;
- both areas have separate storage facilities;
- there are adequate hand disinfection facilities;
- there is no cross-over of clean and dirty instruments;
- there is separate equipment for each area;
- the staff work in either—never in both.

Storage in the SSD

After they have been processed, the sterile packs should be stored in well-ventilated, clean stores ready for dispatch to the wards. Collection should be regular and there should be a written record of receipt and delivery. This helps monitor the use and loss of instruments.

At the North Middlesex Hospital, the sterile services are supplied by a centralized unit that caters for four large health districts. The system is based on an initial ward stock, which is replaced when the label from a used pack is returned to the SSD. However, should extra supplies be required, a requisition form is used and a record of the order is kept; this reduces wastage.

Whatever system is being considered, it is important to keep track of equipment usage and losses.

SSD staff facilities

- All SSD staff should be provided with adequate protective clothing (e.g. heavy-duty gloves, plastic aprons, and eye protection if manual cleaning is undertaken). Overshoes and masks are not necessary.
- SSD staff should be immunized against hepatitis B and an accurate record of all immunizations should be kept by the Occupational Health Department.

- All staff should receive formal training and lectures on the prevention of sharp injuries and the procedure to be followed should an accident occur (see Occupational Health, p. 170).
- There should be policies for handling sharps, inoculation accidents, spillage of body fluids, and accidental splashing with reagents used in the SSD.
- Adequate changing and rest facilities should be provided.
- Adequate handwash facilities must be provided.

Processing instruments

Cleaning

All equipment should be cleaned in the SSD. Equipment requiring sterilization must be cleaned thoroughly before the sterilization/disinfection process. Equipment that is heavily soiled with blood, faeces, and other body fluids is difficult to clean properly. It is not customary for all such soiled equipment to be autoclaved or thoroughly cleaned before handling, to reduce the risk from blood-borne disease. However, where this practice is carried out it poses the problem of cleaning baked-on dirt, which, with inadequate cleaning equipment, can be an extremely laborious process. It is best to clean the instruments carefully and thoroughly before autoclaving.

Mechanical cleaning

Most modern SSDs are automated and there is minimal handling of dirty equipment by staff. The equipment is place in trays ready for washing:.

- *Washing machine.* This gives a cold rinse, followed by a hot wash at 71 °C for 2 minutes. A 10-second hot water rinse at 80–90 °C is followed by drying at 50–75 °C by heater or fan.
- *Washer/disinfector.* This is used for anaesthetic equipment. It runs a 45-minute cycle of washing and cleaning plus a 2-minute cycle with water at 80–100 °C and a detergent solution.
- *Ultrasonicator.* This is a sophisticated, expensive but extremely efficient piece of equipment. It uses high-power output of 0.44 W/cm^{-3} and dislodges all organic matter.

Manual cleaning

Manual cleaning is necessary when:

- mechanical cleaning facilities are not available;
- delicate or difficult instruments have to be cleaned;
- complex instruments need to be taken apart to be cleaned;
- small or narrow-necked jugs and bowls are to be cleaned.

Hand-cleaning must be done with extreme caution (Fig. 4.1). The staff should follow the set procedure:

- Wear heavy-duty rubber gloves, plastic apron, and eye protection.
- Soak the instruments in hot water containing a foaming agent and detergent.
- Drain the water carefully and separate the instruments, and ensure the sharp ends are away from the handler.

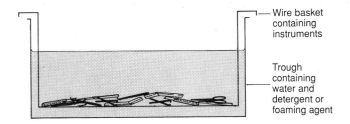

Wire basket containing instruments

Trough containing water and detergent or foaming agent

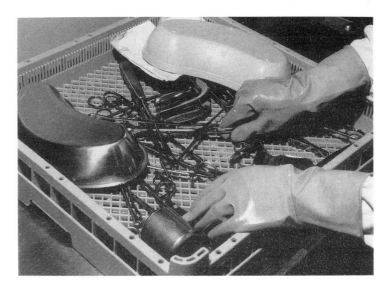

Fig. 4.1 Manual cleaning of instruments.

- Wash the instruments gently. Use a good soft brush if they are delicate and placed a high-pressure jet to clean the inside of hollow needles and tryphines.
- Place the washed instruments on a tray.
- Wrap the tray and place in an autoclave tray prior to sterilization.
- Label clearly.

In units where automated washers are not available a deep container, e.g. a bucket or trough, containing a wire-mesh basket can be filled with hot water and detergent, the instruments placed in the wire basket, agitated for 3–5 minutes, and then lifted out. The basket is overturned on to a table or tray to separate the instruments prior to washing, packing, and autoclaving (Fig. 4.1). This system may be used in operating theatres to reduce contamination.

Sterilization

The different types of sterilization are summarized in Table 4.7.

Heat sterilization

Heat is the most reliable method of sterilization. Most vegetative organisms are killed between 65 and 100 °C by coagulation of their body proteins. However, some organisms, e.g. *Enterococcus faecalis* (72 °C for 3 minutes) and some viruses, are heat-resistant, and spores such as *Clostridium tetani* require temperatures in excess of 100 °C.

Dry heat Hot air ovens are electrically heated by a fan and are fitted with a thermometer and a chart recorder. Items should be wrapped in craft paper or aluminium foil. The sterilization cycle is:

- heat to the required temperature (160—180 °C);
- hold at this temperature for a set period (holding time);
- allow to cool (cooling period).

Dry heat sterilization is suitable for:

- solids;
- non-aqueous liquids;
- closed cavities;
- fine instruments (e.g. optical equipment);

Table 4.7 Methods of sterilization and disinfection

Process	Method	Use
Sterilization		
moist heat	Autoclave	Most common for heat-stable equipment
dry heat	Hot air oven	Fluids and delicate instruments
physico-chemical	Low-temperature steam ± formaldehyde	Heat-sensitive equipment
chemical	Ethylene oxide	May be used (with extreme caution) for heat-sensitive equipment. Use in carefully controlled condition
radiation	Gamma irradiation	Industrial use only
Disinfection		
boiling pasteurizers	Use at 80 °C	Obsolete. Not for surgical instruments
low-temperature steam	Use at 60–80 °C	Heat-sensitive equipment—not commonly used
glutaraldehyde (2%)	3 minutes	Fibre optics
	20 minutes	Gastroscope
	1 hour	Bronchoscope *Mycobacterium tuberculosis*

- glass;
- metal;
- hollow needles;
- heat-stable powders;
- waxes;
- petroleum jelly.

It is unsuitable for rubber, plastics, combustible substances, and glycerol. Its disadvantages are:

- uneven heat distribution in the oven results in a marked temperature variation (up to 60 °C);
- it is a long sterilization cycle.

Radiant heat, such as infra-red and microwaves, may be used for glass syringes, but is not common.

Moist heat Moist heat makes use of gaseous water (steam), which can penetrate and kill bacteria at temperatures lower than those required with dry heat (Table 4.8). Steam sterilization (using autoclaves) is the most common form of sterilization and the steam is often obtained from the boiler room, although it may require modification before it can be used in the autoclave. Once installed, autoclaves are easy to maintain, versatile, economical to run, and efficient.

Table 4.8 Types of steam sterilizers]

Items processed	Temperature of steam (°C)	Types
Wrapped articles	134–138	Mechanical
Wrapped articles	121–126	Downward displacement
Unwrapped articles	132–134	Downward displacement
Bottled aqueous liquid	115–121	Downward displacement
Dressings, rubber, wrapped and unwrapped articles, bottled aqueous liquid	134	Prevacuum

Steam penetrates best when air has been removed. The methods for air removal are:

- mechanical;
- downward displacement;
- pulse prevacuum (the most common method).

The moisture content of the steam is very important. Steam that is under- or oversaturated cannot penetrate the contaminating organisms effectively and the packs of equipment remain wet and non-sterile:

- Saturated steam. The optimum conditions for steam sterilization occur when the steam is saturated (relative humidity = 100 per cent and evaporation and condensation take place at an equal rate). Saturated steam has a high heat content and penetrates the contaminating organisms well. The packs of equipment should come out of the autoclave dry.

- Superheated steam (relative humidity < 100 per cent) is less efficient than saturated steam and may be the result of an overheated steam jacket, pressure reduction in the steam supply or absorption of steam by dehydrated textiles. It is not an effective sterilizing agent.

- Wet steam (relative humidity > 100 per cent) carries droplets of water (from condensation) and is usually the result of poor insulation. It is a poor sterilizing agent, preventing penetration of the contaminating organisms and drying.

It is vital that these differences between the types of steam are understood by the engineers and SSD managers—WET PACKS MUST BE CONSIDERED NON-STERILE.

Blood and tissue reduce the penetration, and therefore the sterilizing effect, of steam. All instruments requiring sterilization must be cleaned.

Steam penetrates contaminating organisms best at a neutral or acid pH.

The most common method for sterilizing of heat-stable instruments and fluids is pressure steam sterilization. The steam supply to the jacket and chamber must come from a common source and gauges are essential to monitor the process. The temperature and saturation of separate steam sources could not be controlled as effectively and differences would result in 'cold spots', which would affect the penetration of the steam.

The sterilization cycle   The sterilization cycle includes:

1. warming the chamber;
2. vacuum extraction;
3. pre-steam penetration time;
4. steam penetration time;
5. holding time;
6. cooling time.

4 + 5 = the sterilization time

These stages should be clearly visible on a temperature recorder, which is usually a dual pen recorder showing the temperature of the chamber and the jacket.

New EEC regulations may modify the standards of autoclave testing and the requirements for SSD.

A common problem is the sterilization of the steam trap, which collects the condensate from the chamber. Rerouting the steam from the jacket to the trap can overcome this problem, but is not routinely indicated.

Ethylene oxide

Ethylene oxide can be used to sterilize most articles that can withstand temperatures of 50–60 °C. However, it should be used under carefully controlled conditions (given in the Health and Safety Guidelines) because it is extremely toxic and explosive. Although it is very versatile and can be used for heat-labile equipment, fluids, and rubber, etc., a long period of aeration (to remove all traces of the ethlyene oxide) is required before the equipment can be distributed.

Low-temperature steam formaldehyde

Steam formaldehyde requires careful use. It is a very versatile method of sterilization but conventional steam sterilization is preferable. Unlike ethylene oxide, low temperature steam formaldehyde requires a long aeration period before the equipment can be used.

Tests of sterilization

To ensure that sterilization has been successful the process of sterilization (and not the end product) is tested. If the system works and runs satisfactorily, the equipment and instruments being sterilized do not need to be tested. Any failure highlighted by the tests casts doubt on the sterility of the equipment. The batch should be recalled and no further sterilization should be done until the fault has been rectified and the system has retested satisfactorily.

Physical tests

Physical tests ensure that the equipment is working properly before the process of sterilization starts:

- *Charts and gauges.* Observations of the temperature charts, particularly the holding time and pressure readings, should be taken at least three times during the sterilization stage to ensure that there is no marked difference between the chamber and jacket temperatures. All recorder charts must be kept for at least a year and should be available for inspection by the engineers and the IC team in the event of an outbreak of infection (Fig. 4.2).

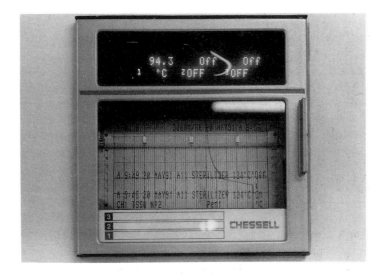

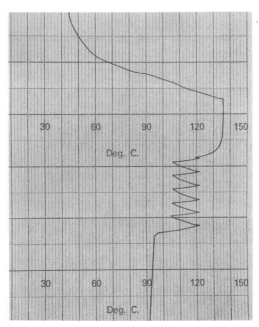

Fig. 4.2 A temperature chart recorder and chart showing the sterilization cycle with the warming up of the chamber, the holding time, pulsed air, and the cooling time.

- *Leak rate test.* This text is performed during the drying stage, when all parts of the sterilizer are hot. The chamber is evacuated to 80–90 kPa below atmospheric pressure. There should be an increase of not more than 133 Pa (1 mmHg) per min. This test should be performed at least weekly on pre-vacuum steam sterilizers.

- *Thermocouple tests.* Several leads are introduced into the chamber, the drains and the items to be sterilized. These record the temperatures in various parts of the autoclave and allow any major variation in temperature to be noted. The chamber must be air-tight during this exercise. This text should be done monthly.

- *Air removal.* Steam cannot penetrate if pockets of air are left in the chamber. A test for air removal uses Bowie–Dick autoclave tape (Fig. 4.3). A cross should be made on a sheet of steam-penetrable paper, which is placed in the centre of a standard test pack of cotton towels. The sterilization stage is limited to 3.5 minutes. The sheet is then inspected for a uniform change of colour, which will indicate steam penetration. A recent alternative, which works on the same principle, is the Lantor cube, which is available in 1228 autoclave test pack (3M). This comes ready packed and is easier to use than the paper.

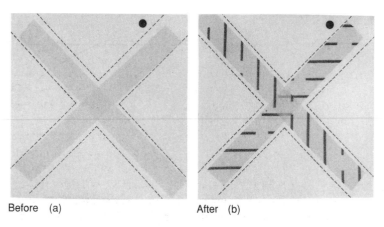

Before (a)   After (b)

Fig. 4.3 The Bowie–Dick test showing the uniform change in the temperature tape before and after a sterilization cycle.

Chemical tests

Chemical indicators are sold as dye strips or tubes containing fluids or granules that change colour at different temperatures. A change of colour occurs when a particular temperature is reached, irrespective of the holding time.

These indicators are used internally, placed where steam or temperature take longest to reach, or externally in the form of strips or tapes on the outside of the packs to distinguish sterilized from non-sterilized packages. They should always be used in conjunction with another testing device because they may change colour before the holding time is over (i.e. before sterilization is complete). They should not be used as the only means of testing sterility.

Examples of chemical indicators include Browne's tube (tubes of coloured fluid), which is used for steam sterilization and hot air sterilizers; Diack Vac Controls (pellets in sealed tubes) and sachets containing a substance that changes colour in such a way as to allow the extent of under-or overexposure to be measures. Sachets containing an acidified solution of magnesium chloride and a pH indicator have also been used.

Chemical indicators are available for testing ethylene oxide, dry heat, steam, and formaldehyde processes. There is no official standard for chemical indicators at present.

Biological tests

Standardized preparations of bacterial spores (strips carrying 10^4–10^6 dry spores) can be placed amongst the equipment to be sterilized. After the sterilization process the strips are placed in a broth that supports aerobic growth and incubated for 7 days at 37°C for *Bacillus subtilis* var. *niger* and 56°C for *Bacillus stearothermophilus*. The end result should be 'total kill'.

Good microbiology facilities and anaerobic culture methods are required for this system, as contamination of the broth cultures can be high in unskilled hands. The expiry date and storage of the spore strips are very important, as inviable spores may falsely indicate sterility. As sterilized equipment cannot be released until the results from the spore strips are available, most SSDs have replaced this test with more sophisticated and faster methods where the spores are supplied in broth containing test tubes and can be incubated in the SSD in special incubators. It is still used in industrial processing, particularly where ethylene oxide and gamma radiation are used. If used for steam sterilization, the text must be performed in conjunction with other, more reliable tests.

Recycling

Recycling equipment is a complex and emotive subject and, in countries with minimal resources, is closely aligned with financial limitations and implication. The law on recycling differs from county to country and law of Good Manufacturing Practice and product liability have resulted in a serious re-evaluation of recycling equipment and the legal implications thereof. All that can be offered here are general guidelines and points to be considered before embarking on a recycling policy.

Why is equipment recycled?
Major reasons for recycling equipment include:

- lack of finances;
- shortage of an assured and regular supply of equipment, especially disposables;
- cost to the hospital of replacing disposables;
- cost to the patient (when disposables are added to the patient's bill);
- problems with delivery. By the time some consignments of equipment arrive the packaging may be damaged or the expiry date may have passed.

The main reasons for recycling are usually cost and shortage of supplies. Recycled equipment falls into three main categories:

- disposable sterile items that have been opened in error;
- used disposable items;
- disposable items that have passed the expiry date.

Formulating a recycling policy
The main points to consider when formulating a recycling policy are:

- *Is the procedure safe?* The ICC must ensure that the procedures available for recycling are monitored and that the end products are sterile. There should be no doubt regarding safety.
- *Is there a genuine cost-saving?* The amount of time and manpower required to meet the required standards of sterility may be more costly than bulk purchase of disposable items. It is sometimes cheaper in the long term to buy non-disposable items that can be safely recycled by autoclaving or other methods of heat sterilization.
- *Is the sterilization/disinfection process effective for that piece of equipment?*
  —are there adequate quality control measures for the end product?
  —are there adequate methods to test the systems employed in recycling?
  —is there any deterioration of the item processed?
  —is there an alteration in the chemical nature of the item which may lead to side-effects in the patient?
- *Is it legal?* Most manufacturers' guarantees will be invalid if a product intended for single use has been recycled. There are important medical and legal implications related to this.
- *Is it ethical?* Is the process justifiable? The acid test here must be whether you would use a recycled urinary catheter, or other recycled equipment, on your own family and friends.
- *What are the manufacturer's instructions on reprocessing?*
- *Can the equipment be cleaned effectively?* Fine- or narrow-bore needles and catheters are difficult to clean and should not be recycled.
- *What is the effect of reprocessing on the equipment?* It is important to know whether there are changes in the chemical composition of the equipment and/or the leaching of altered and toxic chemicals that may adversely effect the patient. Equally, consider the effect of the chemical used during the sterilization process, e.g. ethylene oxide.
- *How many recycling processes will the equipment stand?* If it can only withstand two or three cycles, the effort may not be worth it.

Recycling single-use equipment
The only items of single-use equipment that should be recycled, subject to the considerations given above, are:

● solid metal articles, e.g. stainless steel;

● rubber, latex, and similar materials;

● electrodes.

Items that should not be recycled are:

● fine-bore invasive equipment, e.g. needles and cannulae;

● urinary catheters for general use;

● wound dressings, bandages, and cotton wool;

● administration sets.

The recycling process
The recycling must take place in an SSD and should follow the sterilization procedure given on page 60. A comparison between single-use and recycled equipment is presented in Table 4.9.

Summary

● Establish a Sterile Services Department (SSD).

● Follows the suggested SSD procedure (p. 60) in:
—the ward;
—the SSD.

● All equipment should be cleaned in the SSD, either:
—mechanically;
—manually.

● Sterilization is usually by steam.

● Sterilization equipment should be tested regularly.

● Equipment should be recycled ONLY if:
—the process is safe;
—sterilization is effective;
—recycling is cost-effective.

Table 4.9 Comparison of the advantages and disadvantages of single-use and reuse of equipment

Item	Advantages		Disadvantages	
	Single use	Reuse	Single use	Reuse
Solid surface instruments		Cost-effective	Cost-impractical	Skilled labour required to clean
Heat-labile instruments		Cost-effective	Cost-impractical	Technical problems Needs skilled labour
Clinical devices, e.g. urinary, intravenous catheters	Adheres to the manufacturer's guarantee No risk of cross-infection	Cost-effective Increased user availability	Cost-impractical Availability of supply—possible shortages	Difficult to clean Labour-intensive
Anaesthetic equipment	Adheres to the manufacturer's guarantee No risk of cross-infection	Cost-effective (?) Equipment always in use	Cost (?)	Labour-intensive Technical problems
General equipment	No processing problems	Cost-effective (?)	Cost (?)	Labour intensive
Dressings	No processing problems	Increased availability of dressings Cost-effective (£)	Cost(?)	Time-consuming Wasteful
Linen	Improved bacteriological barriers	Cost-effective (?)	Cost (?)	No bacteriological barrier Need a laundry barriers Losses

Antibiotic policies

It is difficult to formulate a general antibiotic policy because:

- bacterial populations are different in every hospital;
- antibiotic resistance patterns differ;
- clinical choice varies;
- the availability of antibiotics between countries and hospitals;
- the costs of antibiotics (to the hospital and patient) vary;
- the route of administration of antibiotic varies;
- medical and nursing levels affect the route of administration.

It is therefore best to discuss principles rather than specific regimes.

General principles

- Which patient diagnostic group is the antibiotic policy for?
- Are the antibiotics for prophylaxis or therapy?
- What antibiotics are available?
- Which antibiotics share the same clinical efficacy, safety, and routes of administration?
- What effect will the antibiotics have on the bacteria colonizing the patient's gut and on the bacteria in the hospital environment?
- Have the clinicians been consulted and asked for their views on the proposed antibiotic policy?

Formulating an antibiotic policy

- List the indications for which antibiotics are required.
- List the categories of antibiotic, e.g. prophylaxis or therapy.
- List the antibiotics that are similar in spectrum, safety, and pharmacokinetics. the list of antibiotics used for all clinical indications can usually be rationalized to 18–20 antibiotics.
- Draft an antibiotic policy.
- Discuss the draft policy with the clinicians.
- When the policy has been agreed, inform the Microbiology Department and the Pharmacy.

- Enter the policy in the hospital formulary.
- Review the policy periodically.

Antibiotic usage

Antimicrobial agents are used to prevent infection and to treat patients with proven or suspected infection. The aim is to administer a cost-effective and safe dose of antibiotic, which eliminate the infecting, or potentially infecting, organisms.

Antibiotics should be prescribed carefully. Over-use results in resistance—not only to the antibiotics prescribed, but often to those in other classes or groups. Resistance renders the antibiotics ineffective.

The choice of antibiotic

The choice of the particular antibiotic to be used should depend on:

- The spectrum of antibacterial activity.
- Safety (direct and indirect interaction with other drugs).
- Purpose—is the drug for prophylaxis or for therapy? Is it for targeted or empirical therapy? (see below)
- What is the proposed route of administration?
- Cost—is there an equally effective but cheaper alternative?

Prophylaxis

Prophylactic antibiotics are mainly used during surgery (and other invasive procedures) where maximum blood (and tissue) levels of antibiotic are required. There is no benefit to starting prophylaxis days or weeks before the operation—this can result in resistance and is a waste of resources:

- A single (or maximum of three) dose(s) of prophylactic antibiotic should be administered, starting at the induction of anaesthesia.
- Prophylaxis should not continue beyond 24 hours. Antibiotics used after this period should not be considered prophylactic and, if continuation of therapy is required, should be prescribed separately.

The choice of antibiotic is personal but a β-lactam, either a penicillin or a cephalosporin, with or without an aminoglycoside, is usual. Metronidazole may be added if anaerobes are expected. To reduce the possibility of antibiotic resistance during prophylaxis it is sensible to choose antibiotics that will probably not be considered for therapy. However, continuation of the same antibiotic into therapy is quite acceptable provided that the usage and cover have been rationalized.

Therapy

Empirical therapy

This is based on a 'best guess' antibiotic for the suspected organism and its predicted antibiotic sensitivity patterns. Knowledge of local antibiotic sensitivity patterns is useful so that prescribing is not based on publications from other countries, which may not always be applicable.

The range of antibiotics is broad and a combination of two or more may be used initially. This may be reduced to one when the bacteriology results become available.

Targeted therapy

This is used when the bacteriology results are available before treatment or when the range of possible pathogens is limited, e.g. in meningitis. Advice from a clinical microbiologist or infectious disease consultant, with an understanding of the subject is helpful.

Topical antibiotics

The antibiotics used for topical application are also used parenterally. Topical antibiotics should therefore be prescribed carefully, for the following reasons:

- Over-use may result in antibiotic resistance.
- Antibiotic-resistant bacteria may be spread through the hospital (via skin scales, direct contact or in the air).
- Secondary bacterial colonization can occur.
- The antibiotic dosage cannot be controlled.
- Side-effects can occur. The exceptions to this are: (i) ophthalmic preparations containing antibiotics, where the problem of side-

effects seems to be much reduced, although side-effects with chloramphenicol eye drops have been documented; and (ii) mupirocin (Bactroban) ointment which is used to eliminate methicillin-resistant *Staphylococcus aureus* (MRSA). Although plasmid-mediated resistance has been reported, it does not yet appear to be a major problem.

- Topical antibiotics in hospital practice are not recommended.

Rationalizing the use of antibiotics

The use of antibiotics is best controlled via the Drugs and Therapeutics Committee or an Antibiotic Users Committee. Decisions on whether to include particular antibiotics in the hospital formulary should be made only after informed and rational discussion. The IC doctor should be active in making this decision and should provide information relevant to deciding the antibiotic policies. Any changes in antibiotic policy should be referred to the Drugs and Therapeutics Committee and all antibiotic policies should be subject to periodic review.

Only essential antibiotics should be stocked in the Pharmacy and one or two from every group should be available in the formulary. These then need to be categorized into:

- Ward stock, which is freely available for use by all staff (including the junior staff).
- Controlled stock, which is for use only after advice from senior medical staff.
- Restricted stock, which is for use only after consultation between the senior consultant and the clinical microbiologist or infectious diseases specialist (the IC doctor).

Controlling antibiotic usage

A review of antibiotic policies should be considered when there is:

- A change in antibiotic resistance patterns.
- A change in the function of the unit, e.g. new operations being performed or new units being opened.
- New consultant staff who are used to a different policy.
- The introduction of new antibiotics onto the market.

- Pressure from medical representatives to change.
- A price increase for current drugs.

The first two are probably the most valid reasons for reviewing antibiotic policy.

If a new antibiotic is introduced onto the market, it should replace an existing one in the same group, unless it is a completely new class of antibiotic, in which case it should be included in the formulary after consultation with the medical and pharmacy staff and when the indications for its use have been established.

An on-call service for advice on antibiotic therapy by the infectious diseases physician and/or the clinical microbiologist helps to reduce wastage and inappropriate use of antibiotics.

A further means of controlling antibiotic prescribing is by **restrictive reporting**. This means that, although a range of antibiotics may be tested against a particular bacterial isolate, only those that have been agreed in the antibiotic policy will be reported. If the organism is resistant to these (first line) antibiotics, then further antibiotic sensitivities may be reported.

An example of an antibiotic policy

To illustrate the points made in this chapter, Table 4.10 shows an example of an antibiotic policy in use in the North Middlesex Hospital in 1991. This table is an example only—policies will differ according to availability, finance, etc.

Summary

- When formulating an antibiotic policy, consider:
  —the indications for which antibioties are required;
  —which antibiotics are to be included in the policy. Rationalize these into:
  - ward stock;
  - controlled stock;
  - restricted stock.
- Use prophylactic antibiotics only when necessary—overusage results in resistance.
- Review antibiotic policy regularly.

Table 4.10 An example of an antibiotic policy (the North Middlesex Hospital, 1991)

Antibiotic	Route of administration
Ward stock (for use by all staff)	
benzyl penicillin, amoxycillin	i.v./oral
flucloxacillin/cloxacillin	i.v./oral
gentamicin	i.v./i.m.
co-trimoxazole	oral
erythromycin	i.v./oral
cefuroxime	i.v.
metronidazole	oral/p.r.
Restricted used (for use after consultation with senior staff)	
piperacillin (ureido penicillin)	i.v.
chloramphenicol	i.v./oral
co-amoxy clavulanate (Augmentin)	oral/i.v.
fusidic acid	oral/i.v.
clindamycin	oral/i.v.
tetracycline	oral/i.v.
metronidazole	i.v.
Controlled use (for use only with a consultant's signature)	
ceftazidime	i.v.
amikacin	i.v.
ciprofloxacin	oral/i.v.
teicoplanin	i.v.
rifampicin (other than for *Mycobacterium tuberculosis*)	
Other antibiotics that do not appear in the formulary but that may be requested by a consultant	

i.m., intramuscular; i.v., intravenous; p.r., per rectum.

Part 3
Dealing with infection

5. The infected patient

Investigating infection

- All specimens for bacteriological examination should be fresh and sent in sterile containers to the Microbiology Department as soon as possible after collection. The results of bacteriological examination depend on the quality of the specimen. *If specimens are taken in non-sterile containers, or after antibiotic therapy has been started, the results may be inaccurate and/or inconclusive.* A specimen collection system exists in most hospitals and usually takes place twice a day. It is often worthwhile taking urgent specimens directly to the laboratory and speaking to the laboratory staff.

- Most hospitals have an on-call service for dealing with emergency specimens and with specimens that cannot be duplicated, e.g. cerebrospinal fluids, pleural fluids, intra-abdominal fluids or any deep pus. This service is expensive and should not be misused.

- Specimens taken out-of-hours should be kept under optimum conditions until they can be taken for examination. Blood cultures should be kept in a small incubator at 37°C, sputum and urine should be kept in a refrigerator and wound swabs should be kept at room temperature.

- The Microbiology Department should give speedy, accurate, and reliable results, and assist the clinician in confirming the diagnosis.

General principles

- Specimens should be taken *before* starting antibiotic therapy whenever possible. This will result in an increased pathogen isolation rate and reduces the number of repeat specimens required to reach a diagnosis—it ultimately more cost-effective. However, antibiotic therapy need not be delayed until the results are available. From the patient's point of view, early testing of specimens allows earlier targeting of antibiotic therapy, reduces the number of days in hospital and is cheaper.

- Specimens should be put into clearly labelled, leak-proof sterile pots. High risk specimens should be labelled as such.

- Specimens should be accompanied by a request form, which should show the patient's name, age, sex and hospital number, if available. This should be completed with a ball-point pen, stating the name of the requesting doctor, contact number, return destination for the results, the antibiotics the patient is receiving or has just completed, and the duration of therapy (include the date of commencement). If antibiotic therapy is to be started after the specimen has been taken, state what is to be given, so that if there is a significant isolate, it can be tested against the proposed antibiotics for sensitivity and resistance.

- The form and specimen pot should be put in separate compartments of a leak-proof carrier, so that if there is a leak the form can be saved and a further specimen requested.

- Always send fresh specimens of urine, sputum, and stools for processing—the isolation rates are better. Blood culture specimens must be incubated at 37 °C as soon as possible after collection.

- A sample of pus should be sent for wound infections and abscesses. Wound swabs are sometimes acceptable but the isolation rates of fastidious bacteria, particularly anaerobes, is much better from pus.

- If the specimen is unrepeatable, ask the clinical microbiologist for a more intensive investigation.

  The specimens that should be taken in suspected infections are shown in Table 5.1.

Table 5.1 Types of specimens

Suspected infection/symptomatology	Specimen
Diarrhoea	Stools ($\times$ 3)
	Blood cultures, if indicated
Endocarditis	Blood culture ($\times$ 3)
	Acute serum 10 ml clotted blood (save)
	Urine for microscopy
Hepatitis and HIV	Serology specimens:
	10 ml clotted blood clearly labelled 'high risk'

Table 5.1 (*contd.*)

Suspected infection/symptomatology	Specimen
Infection at the site of i.v. devices	All specimens to be sent in a sterile container
	Whole cannula or i.v. catheter sent in sterile pot
	Insertion site swab
	Blood culture
Infective arthritis	Joint aspirate for bacterial tests
	Blood cultures
Meningitis	CSF in two containers: bacterial and viral
	Blood cultures
Multiply antibiotic-resistant Gram-negative bacilli (see pp. 112–14)	Urine
	Stool
	Swabs from moist skin lesions and any other infected site
	Sputum, if ventilated
Ophthalmic infections	Eye swab for:
	bacteria—
	Chlamydia (neonate)
	viral—transport in viral transport medium
Pelvic inflammatory disease	Blood culture (if patient is pyrexial)
	Endocervical swab for:
	bacteria
	Chlamydia
	Intrauterine device (dry sterile pot)
vaginal discharge	Endocervical swabs for:
	bacteria, e.g. *Trichomonas*
	yeast, i.e. *Candida*
Pyrexia of unknown origin	Blood cultures (× 3 in 24 h)
	10 ml clotted blood (acute serum) repeat serum sample in 2 weeks.
	Urine (× 2 in 24 h)
	Stool (× 3 in 72 h)
	Sputum, if present
	i.v. lines for culture (if removed)
	Others—as appropriate
Respiratory tract infection *Upper RTI*	
epiglottitis	Blood culture (NEVER attempt to take a throat swab)
sore throat	Bacterial: throat swab
	Viral: throat swab into viral transport medium for viral culture

Table 5.1 (*contd.*)

Suspected infection/symptomatology	Specimen
Respiratory tract infection (*contd.*)	
Upper RTI (*contd.*)	
whooping cough	Perinasal swab
	Cough plates (fresh medium)
pleural fluid	Fluid: bacterial, viral and
	tuberculosis
	Blood cultures, if indicated
Lower RTI	
pneumonia or chronic	Blood culture ($\times$ 2)
respiratory disease	Sputum (fresh) ($\times$ 2)
	10 ml clotted blood for viral screen
Screening for methicillin-resistant	Swabs from nose, hairline, groin/
Staphylococcus aureus (see p. 109)	perineum, any skin lesion, other
	infected sites
	Urine, if catheterized
Skin rashes	Scrape/vesicular fluid for electron
	microscopy
	Skin swab in viral transport medium
	Stool for virus isolation
	Gargle/throat swab in viral transport
	media
	Clotted blood ($\times$ 2 taken 2–3 weeks
	apart)
Tuberculosis	
respiratory	Sputum ($\times$ 3)
renal	Early morning specimen of urine
Urinary tract infection	Urine (fresh):
	midstream and catheter specimens
	supra-pubic aspirate
	bag specimen (neonates)
	Blood cultures (if patient is pyrexial)

Biopsies (e.g. bone, lung, and lymph node) in a dry container. NOT in formalin

Summary

- Always send fresh specimens for examination (if possible) in a sterile container.
- If specimen must be stored before examination, do this at optimum conditions (see p. 81).
- Take specimens before starting antibiotic therapy.
- Always send request form with specimen (see p. 82).

Isolation policies

The aim of isolating a patient is to prevent the spread of communicable diseases and infection caused by multiply antibiotic-resistant bacteria from the patient. Equally, patients with lowered resistance to infection need to be protected from attending hospital staff and from visitors. When formulating an isolation policy, try as far as possible to fit into the working routine of the unit.

Points to consider

There are many considerations to be taken into account when deciding whether to isolate a patient:

- There should be minimal disruption of, and increase in, the medical and nursing workload.
- The cost of providing isolation facilities and protective clothing.
- The routes of transmission.
- Knowledge of the epidemiology of the pathogen. This will allow modifications to clinical practice without risk of spread of infection.
- Are the current isolation practices based on rational policies (or on tradition)?
- Do not isolate the patient for the wrong reasons (e.g. because it is convenient).
- Consider the psychological effects of isolation on the patient before making the decision to isolate.
- Everyone entering and leaving the room must follow the isolation policy.

The essence of a successful isolation policy is to create a barrier (hence the old term 'barrier nursing') between the patient and others, e.g. staff and patients. This is best done by isolating the patient in a single cubicle, or room, depending on the clinical indication. However, if a separate cubicle/room is not available, the patient may be nursed on an open ward provided that the isolation policy is followed meticulously. Although this is the least favourable option, the patient can be accommodated at one end of the ward, close to the wash-hand basin (and sluice). If more than one patient is affected (e.g. in an outbreak) they should be nursed together in one room (cohort isolation) and looked after by dedicated staff.

Transmission of infection

The routes of transmission of infection from infected patients are via:

- hands (the most common route);
- direct contact with contaminated equipment;
- the respiratory tract, spread by droplets;
- environmental factors (dust, fluids) and skin scales (environmental factors contribute when the colonization rates are high and the bacteria are widely dispersed).

Isolation categories

The isolation categories vary from country to country. Most UK hospitals have adopted four categories, and special instruction are given by the IC Team if variations are necessary.

Isolation category A

These infections are spread by:

- hands;
- direct contact with non-sterile equipment, faeces, and body fluids;
- bedpans/urinals.

For example, multiply antibiotic-resistant bacilli; methicillin-resistant *Staphylococcus aureus* (MRSA); hepatitis A, B, C, and V (viral hepatitis); HIV; enteric pathogens; and wet skin lesions—viral and bacterial.

Requirements

- Cubicle—is desirable (and is essential for MRSA).
- Protective clothing—*gloves* and *aprons* are essential. Masks should be used if indicated.

Isolation category B

This category covers infections spread from the respiratory tract via droplets. For example, viruses (e.g. chicken pox, measles, mumps), meningococci, rotavirus, and open pulmonary tuberculosis prior to 48 hours therapy.

Requirements

- Cubicle—is essential.
- Protective clothing—*masks*, *gloves*, and *aprons* should be worn when handling the patient.

Principles for category A and B isolation

All staff (including senior medical staff) and visitors must agree to abide by the protocol and to wear protective clothing as indicated:

- If possible, attend to the isolated patient last, after dealing with all non-infected patients.
- Wash hands thoroughly and dry before and after contact with the patient.
- Dispose of all clinical waste in a colour-coded bag for incineration.
- Wear gloves to help to patient with a bedpan or urinal. Remove carefully and dispose of the contents directly in the sluice or bedpan disinfector. The bedpan or urinal should then be heat disinfected and dried. **BODY FLUIDS AND FAECES SHOULD NOT BE LEFT IN THE SLUICE AREA.**
- Keep all essential items of patient care in the single cubicle with the patient. Alternatively, if separate equipment is not available, decontaminate reliably before using it on another patient (the same principles apply if the patient is nursed on a open ward).
- Discard disposable gloves and plastic aprons after tending the patient (see Protective Clothing Policy, p. 89 if these have been recycled).
- Do not move between patients without decontaminating the hands, without removing protective clothing or with dirty equipment.

Isolation category C (reverse isolations—protective isolation)

The category C patient has to be protected from other patients and the attending staff. Examples are patients with neutropenia, patients on anti-cancer chemotherapy and severely immunocompromised patients, e.g. transplant patients.

Requirements
- Isolation cubicle is essential.
- Protective clothing, sterile mask, gloves, and apron.

Such patients should be isolated with a minimum of dust, dirt, and wet areas, as all are potential sources of resistant bacteria.

The nurse in charge of the patient must be responsible for education the porters, ward attendants, and visitors about the need for isolation. Equally, the medical staff must be educated to realize their responsibilities towards the patients.

Principles for category C isolation
- Attend to the patient before other patients, if possible.
- Wash hands and wear sterile gloves, apron, and mask.
- Discard protective clothing after attending the patient.
- Wash and dry hands.

Isolation category D (strict isolation)

Category D isolation is only found in specialized unit for highly contagious infections such as pulmonary anthrax, rabies, and viral haemorrhagic fevers. Separate, well-thought-out policies are needed to protect staff dealing with these patients.

Requirements
- Cubicle—is essential (and may be replaced with an aplastic bubble that contains the patient and all essential patient-care equipment).
- Protective clothing—plastic aprons, gowns, masks, and eye goggles should be worn.
- Crockery and cutlery—should be disposable. In Asia, banana leaves may be considered.

Principles for category D isolation
- Disposable non-clinical articles should be used and should **NEVER** be recycled.
- All other clinical equipment should be heat sterilized.
- Air-borne contamination and patient-handling should be kept to a minimum.

- Hospital staff and visitors must be made aware of the risks involved when tending such patients.
- Slow viruses are heat-resistant. Disposable items are recommended.

Protective clothing for isolation procedures

The indications for the use of protective clothing for isolation aseptic procedures is uniform but the type and materials available differ, depending on hospital finances, availability, and choice of the users. Recommendations for protective clothing are given in Table 5.2 (clothing for the operating theatre will be covered in the section on Operating Theatres, p. 142).

Masks

Only high-efficiency filter masks have any protective value, providing protection for 10–15 minutes, or as long as they remain dry. Thin paper masks are not protective once they have become moist, which they do very quickly from the moisture in exhaled air. They are a waste of resources. Cotton masks offer no protection and are not recommended.

Indications

- protective isolation;
- strict isolation;
- respiratory precautions;
- aseptic procedures.

Gloves

- Gloves must be well-fitting and appropriate for the intended purpose.
- Non-sterile clean gloves may be used for routine work.
- Sterile gloves should be used for aseptic procedures.
- Recycled gloves may be used with caution but they should not be used when treating neutropenic patients. They are useful mainly for non-sterile ward procedures and can be decontaminated with an alcohol rub for use between patients. They should be discarded in a separate container and sent for washing and autoclaving.
- Latex gloves are preferred for sterile procedures and for recycling.

Table 5.2 Protective clothing

Procedure	Protective clothing					
	Gowns	Aprons	Gloves	Masks	Caps	
Isolation						
standard precautions		✓	non-sterile			
standard precautions (respiratory)			non-sterile	✓		
enteric		✓	non-sterile			
protective	✓	✓	sterile	✓		
Wound care (only if patient is on isolation procedures)	optional	✓	sterile	optional	✓ optional	
All aseptic procedures		optional	sterile	optional		
Catheter bag change, drainage or removal		optional	non-sterile			
Handling of waste (nursing staff)			non-sterile			

Body cover

- Cotton gowns are permeable to water and may be used for respiratory isolation only; these are no longer recommended.
- Plastic aprons are impervious to fluids and are usually disposable, although heavier duty aprons may be recyclable:
  —disposable aprons are essential for enteric precautions but are expensive and cannot be reused effectively;
  —plastic aprons can be reused provided that they can be disinfected by a wash with warm water and detergent and dried. Wipe with 70 per cent isopropyl alcohol between each patient. The inside should be clearly labelled.

Headgear

- Disposable caps, balaclavas or scarves should be used for reverse isolation and in operating theatres.
- Well-fitting cotton caps and scarves may be recycled (by laundering at a high temperature) if disposable ones are not available. Recycled caps must be changed frequently (at least after every shift; in hot countries they may need to be changed more frequently).

Overshoes

These are not recommended.

Terminal cleaning

At the end of a period of isolation, after the patient has vacated the room, the areas should be thoroughly clean before admitting another patient:

- All the surfaces and walls must be washed thoroughly with warm water and detergent and dried (wipe over with a disinfectant if indicated).
- All bed linen, curtains, etc. that is sent to the laundry should be clearly marked 'infected'.
- The bed mattress and pillow should be wiped with warm water and detergent and dried thoroughly. Occasionally, a disinfectant maybe indicated.

- All heat-sensitive items of equipment that are for common ward use should be wiped over with 70 per cent isopropyl alcohol.
- All autoclavable items should be sent to the SSD.
- All disposable items should be discarded in the containers for clinical waste (see Waste Disposal, p. 38).
- The room should be aired and opened for admission after 24 hours.

If the isolation area is a bed on an open ward, then the entire surrounding area up to the next bed, including curtains, should be treated as detailed above. **There is no need to incinerate laundry or other equipment.** The routine sterilization processes should eliminate pathogens.

NOTE: Gas gangrene (*Clostridium perfringens*) is an endogenous infection and the items used for these cases can be adequately sterilized. There is no need to incinerate—it is a waste of resources.

Fumigation

This is no longer recommended for terminal cleaning after an infected case either on the wards or in theatre. Formalin is toxic and has no advantage over the above procedure.

Summary

- Isolation must be considered carefully (see p. 86).
- Patients should be isolated according to the type of infection (see p. 86).
- Staff should take appropriate precautions and follow recommended policy (see p. 86).
- Isolation room/cubicle should be carefully disinfected at the end of the patient stay (see p. 91).

Patients with blood-borne infections

A single policy should be devised to cover clinical entities with a common route of transmission via blood and body fluids. The same policy should apply to patients with:

- HIV;
- hepatitis B, C, non-A non-B;
- syphilis;
- malaria;
- blood-borne viral and bacterial infections.

The policy should assess the risks to the staff and patients and should apply to all departments dealing with blood and blood products, i.e. renal dialysis, operating theatres, the labour ward, the blood transfusion centre, and transplant units (see also Sharps Disposal Policy, p. 40 and Hepatitis B Policy, p. 174). There must be clear policies on:

- screening patients;
- screening staff before they start to work on the unit;
- disposal of sharps and waste;
- protective clothing;
- inoculation accidents and policy;
- sterilization and disinfection.

Other points to be included in the policy are:

- isolation facilities;
- procedure for dealing with spillage of blood and body fluids;
- intravenous procedures;
- risk to staff.

Good practices and adequate staff training should minimize the risk to staff, although extra care is needed with these patients.

Risk assessment

Risk to staff

- from sharps and hollow needles;
- splashing of conjuctivae and mucous membranes with contaminated blood and body fluids;
- heavy contamination of broken skin, e.g. cuts, dermatitis, etc.;
- handling of large quantities of blood and body fluids without protective clothing.

Risk to patients
- use of recycled hollow needles and syringes;
- contaminated blood transfusion;
- heavy soiling of the environment;
- poor ward facilities and cleaning.

Protective clothing

Universal precautions mean that particular high risk procedures are always dealt with using protective clothing, e.g. gloves, aprons, etc.

Countries with a low incidence of blood-borne diseases sometimes practice a two-tier system (protective clothing is used only for known high-risk patients, such as HIV-and hepatitis-B-positive patients). However, a single-tier system (where universal precautions are applied to all patients) should be practised when the incidence is high.

Gloves

Gloves should be made of latex and should fit well. Disposable gloves are recommended *unless* heat disinfection is available. Alcohol disinfection between patients is not recommended because the viruses can become 'fixed' to the latex by the alcohol.

Plastic aprons

These should be worn to protect staff from body fluids. Again, disposable aprons are preferable to recycles ones.

Eye protection

Goggles or some sort of eye protection (visor) should be worn to avoid conjunctival splash contamination. Spectacles are acceptable.

Masks

These are recommended to avoid blood or body fluids splashing into the mouth and nostrils.

Isolation facilities

Single cubicles should be provided only for patients who need high-dependency nursing. If a special ward or unit is available, all patients should be treated as high risk (see Isolation category A, p. 86) and isolation is not necessary.

Spillage of blood and body fluids

Spillages should be dealt with as quickly as possible:

- wear domestic or latex gloves;
- cover the spillage with hypochlorite granules (presept) or paper towels soaked with hypochlorite solution (1000 p.p.m. of available chlorine or 10 000 p.p.m. for heavy soiling);
- allow 2 minutes contact time;
- clear spillage and dispose of as clinical waste;
- wash surface with warm water and detergent;

Sterilization and disinfection

All the pathogens in this category are killed by heat sterilization. Recommended minimum temperatures are:

- $115\,°C \times 30$ minutes or;
- $121\,°C \times 15$ minutes or;
- $126\,°C \times 10$ minutes or;
- $134\,°C \times 3$ minutes.

Ultraviolet light in doses lower than 5×10^3 J/m^2 or gamma radiation below 2×10^5 rads do not eliminate these viruses.

Heat-sensitive equipment (e.g. fibre optics) should be disinfected with 2 per cent glutaraldehyde for at least 10–30 minutes and rinsed thoroughly before use. Heat disinfection ($85\,°C \times 3$ minutes) is also effective.

Disinfectants

Hypochlorites are recommended for surfaces and 2 per cent gluteraldehyde for heat-sensitive equipment.

Intravenous procedures

These must be performed with great care by an experienced practitioner:

- Gloves and plastic aprons should be worn; eye protection is optional.
- A closed system (Vacutainer) is recommended but if a hypodermic needle and syringe must be used the whole unit must be discarded in a sharps container. **DO NOT RESHEATH NEEDLES.**
- Cannulae, hypodermics, and Vacutainers with retractable needles are available for use on high-risk patients. Although these are expensive and cumbersome to use, they greatly reduce the risk of needle-stick injuries.

Collection and transportation of blood from patients

- Perform an absolute minimum of tests on high-risk patients.
- Collect specimens (using a closed system, see above) in secure containers, label clearly and put in a leak-proof bag with request form.
- (Venepuncture should only be performed by an experienced phlebotomist. Double gloves may be worn and a disposable paper towel should be placed beneath the patient's arm to reduce contamination from accidental blood spillage.)
- Any gauze or soiled paper towels should be discarded in the clinical waste bag.
- Transferring the blood to an appropriate container should be done slowly and carefully and without creating an aerosol.
- Needles should not be resheathed but discarded in the sharps container. However, if resheathing is absolutely necessary, use a mushroom device, which holds the cap so the needle can be introduced safely. Alternatively, lay the cap on the table with the closed end against anything that offers resistance and insert the needle carefully—**NEVER** hold the cap while resheathing.

Waste disposal

See page 40.

Staff protection and immunization

- All staff working with category A (hepatitis B, HIV) patients must be immunized against hepatitis B.
- Staff should have adequate training in the care of patients who are HIV- or hepatitis-B-positive and should be aware of the risks involved.
- Clear policies of safety, covering inoculation accidents must be available.
- All inoculation accidents must be reported and documented.
- Frequent lectures are essential to allay fear and promote good morale.

Needle-stick injuries

- If a non-immunized member of staff sustains a needle-stick injury they should be offered hyperimmune gammaglobulin within 48 hours of the injury and a course of hepatitis B vaccination should be started, if the source is Hepatitis B'e'ag positive; if not then Hepatitis B vaccine alone is sufficient.
- If the source is known to be HIV-positive, zidovudine may be administered within 24 hours of exposure and counselling should be offered to the injured member of staff. Zidovudine is reported to delay, but not to prevent, the disease process. It has serious side-effects and its efficacy has yet to be proven.

Special departmental policies

Operating theatres and the labour ward

There has been much discussion recently about the protection of surgeons and staff operating on HIV- and hepatitis-B-positive patients. Recent figures from the USA show that the overall risk of acquiring a blood-borne disease is 0.3 per cent in surgical operations.

Guidelines

The hepatitis B and/or HIV status of the patients should be determined before the operation (the latter is voluntary). The theatre/labour ward staff (and IC Team) should be informed so that appropriate preparations can be made:

- An adequate supply of hypochlorite and a new sharps disposal container should be ordered.

- All disposable items used during the operation (administration sets, i.v. cannulae, etc.) should be disposed of in the sharps container.
- The sharps container should be sealed and disposed of as soon as possible after the procedure.
- All instruments should be sent to the SSD or TSSU after the procedure. They should be clearly labelled as high risk. No attempt should be made to wash the instruments after the procedure.
- Non-disposable items should not be incinerated—they can be sterilized.
- Linen should be sent to laundry marked as 'infected linen'; there is no need for incineration. Pre-packed, disposable, sterile packs may be used, if available.
- All staff should wear protective clothing (see p. 89).
- Keep equipment and staff to a minimum.
- Suction—disposable suction tubing is preferred. Where this is not available send for autoclaving after use.
- Disposal of abdominal swabs:
  —there should be minimal handling;
  —the contaminated (blood-soaked) swabs should be discarded by the surgeon into individual plastic bags; this will facilitate weighing and counting. The swabs can then be discarded. Soaking in a disinfectant such as hypochlorite is not necessary.
- Where possible avoid electrical and other delicate equipment, which is difficult to sterilize.

After the procedure:

- All disposable, incineratable waste should be removed in clearly labelled colour-coded bags.
- Wash surfaces with warm water and detergent.
- Wash walls up to hand height with water and detergent.
- Spot clean blood and body fluid spillage with hypochlorite (see p. 95).
- Send heat-stable equipment for sterilization. Label 'high risk'. Do not soak in bleach.
- Send respiratory equipment for heat- or 2 per cent glutaraldehyde-disinfection (label clearly).

- Wipe large machines (e.g. diathermy and anaesthetic equipment) with warm water and detergent to remove organic contamination. This is sufficient unless heavy soiling has occurred, when they should be wiped over with hypochlorite. Do not allow excessive exposure to hypochlorite—it **corrodes metal**.

Post-delivery care and immunization

- Isolate mother and baby in a cubicle if available and institute enteric precautions (see Category A Isolation, p. 86).
- All babies born to hepatitis B surface antibody positive mothers should be immunized against hepatitis B within 48 hours of birth. If the mother is known to be HBe antigen positive, the baby should also receive hyperimmune gamma-globulin.
- Take blood from the baby when 24 hours old and repeat 3–6 weeks later to confirm hepatitis status, and 3 months later for HIV testing if indicated.
- Wear protective clothing (gloves and disposable gowns) when handling blood and body fluids.
- Protective clothing should be disposed of in a clinical waste bag within the cubicle.
- Place all body fluids (discharge and lochia) in a bag. Label as **CLINICAL WASTE—HIGH RISK** and send for incineration.
- Toilet facilities. If private facilities are available with the cubicle, the bowl should be cleaned and wiped over daily. If facilities are not available then a bedpan should be provided, which should be immediately emptied and disinfected in the bedpan disinfector.
- Send all linen, clothing, etc. to the laundry labelled 'infected linen'.
- Label clearly all investigatory specimens taken from mother and baby.
- Mobile mothers may use communal recreational facilities and tend to their own needs.

Renal dialysis unit

The same basic principles apply to the dialysis unit as to the operating theatre and delivery room:

- Staff should be immunized against hepatitis B before starting work in the unit.

- All patients should be screened and immunized against hepatitis B.
- Disposable tubing and heat-labile equipment are recommended for dialysis.
- The outer surfaces of the renal dialysis machine should be cleaned with warm water and detergent.
- The inside of the machine should be cleaned with 1 per cent chloros (hypochlorite) and rinse thoroughly before further use.
- Disposable filters should be used to prevent contamination with blood.
- Disposable administration lines, dialyser, and needles should be used.
- Equipment to be recycled should be able to withstand autoclave temperatures of 121 °C.

Summary

- A single policy should cover all infectious blood-borne diseases. It should take into account:
  —protective clothing and immunization for staff;
  —isolation;
  —spillages of blood/body fluids;
  —sterilization;
  —i.v. procedure;
  —waste disposal.

6. Outbreaks

Principles of investigating an outbreak

Any increase in the isolation rate of a particular organism, or any clustering of clinical cases should be investigated by the IC team. Infection rates and isolates of particular interest may be monitored by:

- a daily report from the Microbiology Department;
- a prevalence survey of infection;
- notification from the national surveillance centre (the communicable diseases centre), which reports national epidemics.

If an outbreak occurs the aim of investigation is to:

- discover how the outbreak arose;
- treat the infected patients;
- prevent spread of the infection with the minimum of disruption to the patients and staff.

Obtaining surveillance information

Careful surveillance should alert the IC team to possible outbreaks. Suspicion should be raised when:

- A laboratory report of a bacteriology specimen yields an alert organism.
- Two or more patients are found to have an infection attributed to a species not previously documented, particularly if this occurs after a surgical procedure.
- Multiple infections of a similar nature are reported by the clinicians or ward staff.

Following up surveillance information

Single case caused by a nosocomial pathogen

If the surveillance information reveals a new isolate:

- *The IC nurse* should obtain details of the patient and of the source of the isolate from the nurse in charge of the ward. There may have been a breakdown in procedure, or new patient may have been admitted from another hospital. Once the cause has been established, the IC nurse should go over the procedure with the ward staff to reassure them and to ensure that the policy is understood and properly implemented.
- *The IC doctor* should:
  —contact the clinical team responsible for the patient;
  —discuss the problem with the clinicians;
  —warn of the possible implications of the outbreak.
- *The patient* should be dealt with according with established infection control policy.
- No further action, except vigilance, is required.

Two or more cases—potential or actual outbreak

Two or more cases of a nosocomial infection must be dealt with quickly to prevent any further cases. Each case should be investigated fully but with the minimum disruption to the routine. If an outbreak is confirmed, there are several ways of dealing with it, but the most important aspect is communication.

Occasionally, the ward may need to be closed to:

- prevent further spread;
- allow the outbreak to be investigated fully;
- establish the source of the outbreak.

If closure is necessary, the staff must be made fully aware of the consequences and the ward should be reopened as soon as possible.

Guidelines for investigating an outbreak

Investigating a potential outbreak can be very time-consuming and all aspects of the outbreak must be covered during the initial investigation—there may not be another chance.

Step 1—preliminary information about the organism

The IC doctor and nurse should establish:

- is it a known organism with a new antibiotic sensitivity pattern, or a new species not previously isolated?

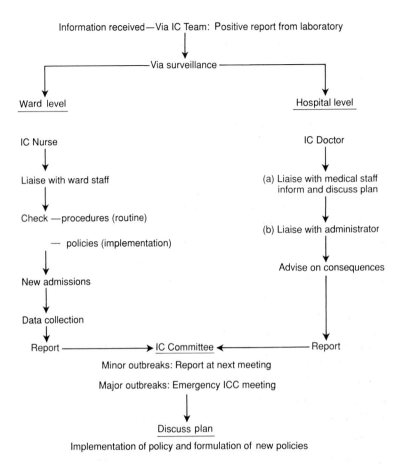

Fig. 6.1 Summary of an outbreak situation.

- has the organism has been isolated previously in any department within the hospital.?
- has it been imported from another hospital?

Step 2—visit the ward

The IC team should visit the ward together to establish whether there have been any breaches in infection control procedure. For example:

- has nursing procedure altered?

- have there been staff shortages?
- is the staff overworked, and consequently taking short-cuts?

This is an opportune moment to review the infection control procedures with the ward staff.

The IC doctor should assess the patient's clinical stage and determine whether the organism has been isolated from a genuine infection from bacterial contamination/colonization of the specimen. It is essential to differentiate between the two. Antibiotics may be necessary if infection is involved, and may be prescribed, after consultation with the clinician in charge of the patient. However, if bacterial contamination is suspected, a further specimen should be taken, to confirm the bacteriological diagnosis. Multiply antibiotic-resistant Gram-negative bacilli isolated from urine are particularly likely to be contaminants.

IC policies should be enforced while awaiting the results of biological examination of the specimen.

Further action

Even if no further action is necessary, the incident should be documented for future reference. Record:

- the patient's name, age, sex, and hospital number;
- the name/number of the ward;
- the name of the consultant in charge;
- the date of admission;
- the procedures that were carried out;
- where the procedures were carried out and when (dates);
- who carried out the procedure;
- what drugs were prescribed, other than antibiotic therapy;
- who prescribed the drugs;
- was therapy changed, and why;
- the patient's current antibiotic therapy and dosage;
- why this antibiotic therapy was started;
- whether the patient was given different antibiotics before the current therapy and, if so, in what dosage and for how long;
- when the pathogen was isolated;

- where the pathogen was isolated from;
- the result from the repeat specimen (if one was taken).

Step 3—liaison with medical staff

- The IC team must inform the medical team in charge of the patient that it is investigating the patient's infection.
- The medical staff should join the IC team on the ward so that an accurate history of the infection can be obtained. For example, where there any changes in medical practice or admissions policy?
- The IC team should take this opportunity to talk to the junior medical staff about the hospital's IC policy and to determine their knowledge of IC procedures. (This is not a court of inquiry, just a means of assessment and communication relating to infection control.)
- Discuss the possible consequences of further cases, should any occur, and the effect that IC measures might have on the running of the ward and on patient care and morale. Some modifications may be necessary but these should not compromise the basic principles of infection. The aim is to stop further cross-infection with the minimum of disruption.
- Discuss the possibility of drastic short-term measures, e.g. ward closures, the effect these might have on further admissions, and the benefits compared with the long-term control of cross-infection. Closing wards is a major (and expensive) step and many clinicians will oppose such a move. It is therefore necessary to consider alternatives, which may take longer but that could be equally successful in the long term. However, cross-infection in highly specialized areas, e.g. orthopaedic wards with implant surgery and cardiac units, can be disastrous.
- The IC doctor should:
  —highlight the long-term consequences of a nosocomial outbreak.
  —Talk about IC policy with the clinicians, who may previously have been less than co-operative—they will probably be more flexible if they feel that help is at hand.
  —Suggest the introduction of IC procedures, such as handwashing, that were previously difficult to implement.

The IC team must be careful not to adopt an air of interrogation. Aggressive behaviour will achieve nothing and will only alienate the medical staff. The IC team is there to help, and not to take over clinical management.

Step 4—inform the administrators

The IC doctor should inform the hospital administrator of the consequences of the outbreak:

- If it becomes necessary to close the ward. Most administrators do not willingly accept the closure of hospital beds because of the financial implications. A suitable alternative, such as a separate ward, opened on a temporary basis to accommodate new admissions, could be considered.
- If any of the IC measures have cost implications. If the ward cannot be closed, the IC doctor must explain the effects the outbreak may have on future admissions to the affected ward, as will as the cost implications of additional antibiotic therapy, nursing time, bed occupancy, repeat surgical procedures, and use of equipment.

An outbreak of a nosocomial infection may have a knock-on effect on the admissions department.

Step 5—report to the ICC

The IC team must report to the ICC so that IC policies and their implementation can be reviewed and modifications suggested, if necessary.

Minor Outbreaks

The report can be made at the next routine ICC meeting.

It may be necessary to call an emergency ICC meeting, which should be attended by:

- the chair of the ICC (usually the IC doctor);
- the IC team;
- the medical and nursing staff in charge of the infected case or ward;
- the hospital administrator.

Once the necessary information relating to the outbreak has been collected, it should be discussed at this meeting. A new policy may be needed to prevent future outbreaks and it is important that all aspects are considered carefully. The IC team should submit an outline plan for discussion and approval, if this is necessary. It is very important to include the medical staff and the hospital administrator in this.

Ward closure

Ward closure is recommended only as an extreme measure, e.g. if there is an outbreak of methicillin-resistant *Staphylococcus aureus* on a high dependency ward, or an incidence of food poisoning.

Procedure

- Close the ward to further admissions.
- Screen all patients and staff.
- Discharge all patients who are fit to go home (on treatment for potential sites of infection/colonization, especially if the outbreak
  is caused by MRSA).
- Keep all other patients in the ward. Do not transfer to another ward—this may further spread the bacterium.
- Use staff who are carriers to look after the remaining patients; their carrier sites should be treated.
- If necessary, open a separate ward for fresh admissions (use uninfected staff).
- Move staff who are found to be negative on screening.
- Isolate the remaining patients (see p. 86) and treat carrier sites.
- Rescreen the isolated patients and their staff.
- When all the patients and staff have been found to be clear, the ward can be cleaned (see p. 91) and reopened.

Further action

The IC team should visit the previously infected ward and assess the situation until satisfied that:

- IC policies are being properly implemented;
- There have been no further cases.

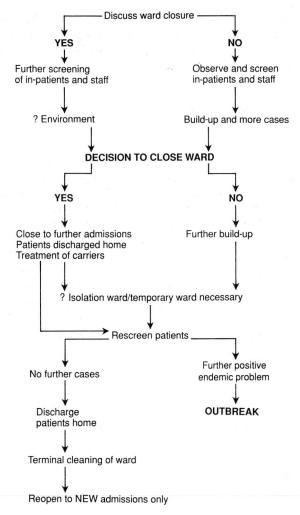

Fig. 6.2 Plan for ward closure during an outbreak.

- The morale of the staff has recovered (most staff feel guilty and responsible for infection and it is important to reassure them regularly).
- The patients' morale has recovered (the upheaval on the ward and isolation of infected patients can be upsetting).
- The infection has not spread to other areas of the hospital.

Recheck hospital practices. If possible, information on the resistance patterns and the prevalence of nosocomial organisms in referring hospitals should be collected, so that an admissions policy can be drawn up.

Methicillin-resistant *Staphylococcus aureus* (MRSA)

Staphylococcal infections are common in hospitals and are usually endogenous. Methicillin resistance is a significant marker for *Staphylococcus aureus* and is best detected by incubating specimens at 30 °C. MRSA is resistant to all cephalosporins, and may be associated with resistance to erythromycin, tetracycline, fucidic acid, and gentamicin. Thus, presently the treatment of choice for MRSA infections is with glycopeptides, e.g. vancomycin or teicoplanin.

The spread of methicillin-sensitive and methicillin-resistant *Staphylococcus aureus* is similar and the mortality rates are no different. However, MRSA poses a particular problem in orthopaedic, intensive care, cardiac surgery, and burns units. This, in terms of morbidity and provision of nursing is high.

Reservoirs of MRSA

nose and groin;
skin lesions;
dust and environment;
linen and bed clothing.

Route of spread

- hands;
- skin scales for excoriating skin lesions;
- air and environment (unusual);
- equipment—clinical and non-clinical (rare).

Control of spread

- Isolation of infected patient(s) in cubicle(s).
- Hand disinfection between patients.

- Gloves when handling patients with wound or skin lesions, urinary catheters, etc.
- Masks are not necessary.
- Do not use the antibiotics to which the MRSA is resistant. The exception is the topical use of mupirocin for the elimination of staphylococci on the skin and nose.
- Always cap the needle (see p. 96) after a syringe has been drawn up with antibiotic and the air bubbles are being released. (An uncapped needle discharges an aerosol of antibiotic when the air bubbles are released and this destroys the commensal bacteria in the nose, providing an opportunity for colonization by MRSA.)
- It may be necessary to close the ward if three or more patients are found to have MRSA. Thorough ward cleaning, laundering of all bed linen and disinfection of equipment (see p. 118) is essential before reopening the ward to new admissions (see Outbreak Investigation, p. 107).

DO NOT TRANSFER INFECTED PATIENTS TO ANY OTHER PART OF THE HOSPITAL EXCEPT TO AN ISOLATION WARD.

Patient screening

Patients on the ward where an outbreak has occurred must be screened, in case the organism has spread.

Screening sites are the nose, groin, axilla, hair line, any wounds or skin lesions, and urinary catheters. Patients receiving antibiotics, especially cephalosporins and steroids, should be included.

All patients being admitted to wards for the elderly should be screened on admission. During an outbreak of MRSA in the community, the author's hospital (the North Middlesex Hospital) first admitted these patients to a cubicle, where they were screened and, if clear, transferred to the open ward. If they would found to be infected, they were kept in the cubicle.

All patients on wards with elderly or high-risk patients should be provided with Irgasan (Cidal soap). Regular use appears to reduce the colonization rate.

If asymptomatic patients are found to be carriers of MRSA, it is worthwhile discharging them from hospital on an anti-staphylococcal protocol (see below). This will reduce the reservoir of MRSA in the community and, therefore, amongst patients being admitted to hospital in the future.

Treatment protocol for MRSA

Nasal carriage for patients and staff

The following 7-day protocol applies to patients and staff colonized with MRSA:

- nasal preparation of:
  —mupirocin (Bactroban) or;
  —chlorhexidine or;
  —naseptin;
- medicated soap (Cidal or Sterzac);
- medicated bath sachets (Sterzac (hexachlorophene), 10 per cent);
- chlorhexidine hairwash (Hibiscrub (100 ml).

Table 6.1 outlines the recommended treatment.

Special instructions for staff who are carriers

- Do not sit on patients' beds.

Table 6.1 Treatment of MRSA nasal carriage

Site	Instructions for treatment
Nares	Apply mupirocin three times a day
Skin	Wash with medicated soap
	Bathe daily with one sachet of medicated bath concentrate
	Powder body with medicated powder
Hair	Wash weekly with chlorhexidine hairwash
Clothes	Change daily and wash in hot water
	Dry clean non-washables and woollens
Bed linen	Change at start of protocol, on day 3 and at end of protocol
Soft furnishings	Clean thoroughly
Carpets	Vacuum thoroughly
Personal items (soft)	Wash or dry-clean at the start of the protocol

- Do not work in any high dependency unit (operating theatre, intensive care unit, or neonatal unit) until clear.
- Staff working on ordinary wards or involved in administration can return to work after three days of starting the anti-staphylococcal protocol with mupirocin, but must be meticulous about personal hygiene and hand disinfection.
- Follow the MRSA protocol for 7 days.
- Clearance swabs should be taken three days after the last application of medication. The results should be available before duty is resumed on a high dependency unit. If carriage has not cleared, further investigation might be necessary.

The IC doctor should be informed if the member of staff (or the patient) is on antibiotics, as these may affect the clearance of MRSA and the protocol may have to be repeated after the course of antibiotics is completed.

Multiply antibiotic-resistant Gram-negative bacilli

One of the major side-effects of broad-spectrum antibiotic usage and advanced invasive medical techniques is the emergence and spread of multiply antibiotic-resistant Gram-negative bacilli (MRGN). These organisms may be intrinsically resistant to the more commonly used β-lactam antibiotics or, more usually, carry anti-biotic resistance plasmids, which can spread not only between the same species, but also to other species. MGRNs are now endemic in most hospital environments and cause great concern to IC teams the world over.

Reservoirs of MRGN

- hands of staff and attendants;
- stools of patients on broad-spectrum antibiotics;
- drains and sinks;
- non-clinical and poorly disinfected clinical equipment;
- open containers of disinfectants;
- bars of soap lying in pools of water.

Routes of spread

MRGNs are spread via:

- hands and non-compliance with hand disinfection procedures;
- bedpans and urinals;
- bed clothes that become contaminated with urine or faeces;
- staff sitting on the beds of colonized patients;
- use of antibiotics that further select for plasmids conferring anti-biotic resistance;
- open containers of contaminated disinfectants and other fluids on the ward.

General principles for control of MRGN bacilli

- Bacterial spread is mainly via hands and contaminated bed pans and urinals:
  - —implement meticulous hand disinfection;
  - —heat-treat bedpans and urinals. Bedpan disinfectors must be operational at all times, at 80°C. Breakdowns should be treated as emergencies;
  - —provide a dedicated bedpan (if possible) for MRGN stool carriers;
  - —ensure that is an adequate supply of gloves and plastic aprons.
- Bed clothing can become contaminated:
  - —do not sit on the patient's bed;
  - —disinfect hands with hand rub immediately after contact with an infected patient.
- Urinary catheters can become colonized:
  - —ensure that an aseptic procedure is used for insertion of catheters;
  - —do not catheterize patients repeatedly;
  - —empty the urinary drainage bag by the tap and wear disposable gloves while doing so. Do not break the circuit and re-connect.
  - —disinfect hands immediately afterwards;
  - —use a separate jug or container for each patient when emptying urinary drainage bags.
- Indiscriminate antibiotic usage increases risk of spread:
  - —restrict antibiotics to necessary use only;

—use antibiotics to which the bacterium is known to be sensitive (ask the IC team for advice if there is any doubt);

—consider using antibiotics where drug resistance is non-plasmid-mediated.

- Disinfectants as a source of MRGN (everything on the ward must be stored DRY):
  —contaminated because of multiple use or left open;
  —soaking of instruments;
  —out of date.

- Heat disinfection of non-clinical equipment is necessary:
  —ensure that the engineers maintain the bedpan disinfectors;
  —ensure that disinfectants are not substituted for heat disinfection;
  —ensure that bedpans, urinals, and bowls are stored clean, inverted, and dry.
  —in the absence of bedpan disinfectors, ensure that bedpans are washed in hot water and dried. Wipe with 1 per cent phenolic if necessary. Wipe with damp cloth to remove disinfectant. Dry.

- Clinical equipment must be sterilized or heat disinfected:
  —ensure that the SSD and TSSU are providing a reliable service and that all heat-labile equipment is properly disinfected.

- Patients transferred between units can spread MRGN:
  —do not transfer patients between wards or hospitals unless it is absolutely essential. If transfer is essential, the IC team should be informed. They will contact the unit receiving the patient to give details of the patient's infection and the necessary precautions.

- Patients with three consecutive clear stools may be returned to the open ward:
  —send stool specimens for clearance—three specimens in a week. Check other sites, such as urinary catheters and skin lesions, for clearance.

7. Design of wards and specialized units

General wards

Most hospital in-patients are treated in wards, which require considerable planning to minimize the risk of cross-infection.

Layout of a ward

The ward layout depends on whether a pre-existing building has been converted, or whether the unit has been purpose-built. There are three main designs:

- *Nightingale wards.* These are dormitory in style, with toilets, bathrooms, sluice areas, etc., at both ends and a nursing station in the centre. There may be a few rooms off the main wards, which are used as treatment rooms, offices, or isolation cubicles. Wash-hand basins are usually at either end of the ward and near the nursing station.
- *Bay wards.* These comprise four-or six-bedded bays, separated by solid or glass partitions, extending on either side of a central nursing station. The toilet and cleaning facilities are usually sited in the centre, opposite the nursing station. Wash-hand basins should be available in each bay.
- *Race-track wards.* These are single-and multiple-bedded units off a quadrangular corridor. The toilet and cleaning facilities are sited in the central area and the nursing station is at the entrance to the ward. Wash-hand basins should be sited in each cubicle or ward area.

Whichever layout is employed, the beds should be at least 2 metres (6 feet) apart, to prevent contact between patients. Close proximity of beds, overcrowding, and even sharing of beds will result in an increase in cross-infection. From an IC perspective, bayed wards are the best, because patients can be contained more easily in smaller, segregated units.

Single cubicles should be included in all newly planned wards. A 40-bedded unit should have at least two such cubicles, preferably with integrated toilet and shower facilities.

Dirty and clean ward areas should be well-demarcated and there should be a separate treatment room for the storage of clean and sterile equipment, and a sluice room for the dirty equipment and the disposal of ward waste, body fluids, etc.

Areas of potential risk
The key word is DRY.

The treatment room
- This must be kept meticulously clean.
- Equipment should be removed immediately after use.
- Containers of fluid should never be left open. This includes cheatle jars filled with disinfectants and containers used for soaking instruments.
- Dressing packages received from the SSD should be stored here, ideally on dry, dust-free racks (moisture will encourage contamination).
- The storage area should be cleaned at least once a month or more, if necessary, with warm water and detergent, dried, and restocked.
- All pre-packed sterile medical and surgical disposable and non-disposable equipment must be checked regularly and returned to the SSD before, or on, the expiry date.
- All equipment must be stored clean and dry.

The sluice room
This should contain:

- a large sink or slop-hopper to dispose of body fluids;
- a bedpan disinfector (80°C × 1 minute) for bedpans, urinals, and urine jugs;
- a rack, with a drip tray, should be provided for clean bedpans and urinals. This should be cleaned daily;
- a hand-wash basin (near the door).

Staff rest-room

This should be separate from the main ward and treatment areas and should contain facilities to prepare food and hot drinks. (The ward sluice room and/or treatment room should not be used to prepare food or drinks.)

Doctors' office

A doctors' office, where the medical staff can write notes and hold case conferences, is essential. It should not contain items of equipment required for patient care—these should be in the treatment room.

Cleaning programme

Warm water and detergent remove 80 per cent of micro-organisms, the majority of which are skin flora and spores, and are quite harmless unless there is a particularly virulent strain of bacterium that is transmitted by air currents. The ward should only be disinfected during an outbreak:

- Damp cleaning (mopping) is recommended. Sweeping disperses dust and bacteria.
- Colour-code the equipment used in the dirty and clean areas of the ward.
- Clean the ward areas daily or more frequently, according to the climatic conditions and the levels of dust in the atmosphere.
- The cleaning should start in the clean areas of the ward and progress to the dirty areas (including the toilets, which should be last).
- The floors should be mopped with warm water and detergent. The water should be changed frequently. Dry the floors.
- Wash the bucket out after use and store dry.
- Mops should be laundered daily in very hot water and detergent, or in a washing machine (if available) and dried thoroughly. Do not leave a wet mop in a bucket—this encourages Gram-negative bacilli.
- Ward surfaces, rails, bedsteads, etc. should be damp-dusted. Do not allow the surfaces to remain wet. No disinfectant is necessary.

- Baths should be washed with warm water and detergent and dried.
- Toilets must be cleaned regularly and left dry. Toilet floors must be dried thoroughly.

Staff health

(See Occupational Health, p. 170).

- All open skin lesions or abrasions must be covered with a waterproof dressing.
- Staff with rashes or diarrhoea, or those who have been in contact with family members with rashes or diarrhoea must report to the Occupational Health Department.

Equipment and patient-care articles

An essential aspect of patient care is to reduce cross-infection between patients and between patients and staff via clinical and non-clinical equipment or fomites.

Where possible, alternatives have been suggested, although many situations have no alternative.

General-use articles

Washing bowls

These must be washed thoroughly between each patient and stored inverted to dry. Use fresh water and towels for each patient.

Bedpans and urinals

- Non-sterile (or recycled) gloves should be worn to empty the bedpan and its contents directly into the bedpan disinfector. *Alternatively*, put down the sluice or toilet.
- Wash thoroughly with warm water using a brush and detergent to remove all visible signs of organic contamination. Dry.

Methods for disinfecting bedpans (in order of preference)

1. Dispose of bedpan contents and disinfection is in a bedpan disinfector, which functions at no less than 80°C for 1 minute.

2. Wash in hot water and detergent. Store inverted in the sun to dry.
3. Wash thoroughly to remove all visible contamination. Dry. Wipe over with 1 per cent phenolic only if essential. Wipe again with wet paper towel. Dry. This is the least satisfactory method and is subject to much abuse.

Do not soak bedpans or urinals in disinfectant—it is unnecessarily expensive and increases the risk of cross-infection with Gram-negative bacilli, which are usually multiply antibiotic-resistant.

Towels, soap, hairbrushes, shaving brushes, razors, etc.

All these items should be for individual use only and should never be shared.

Crockery and cutlery

- Each patient should have an individual set, either provided by the hospital or brought from home.
- Wash crockery and cutlery in very hot water (> 60 °C) and detergent.
- Disposable crockery is necessary only in cases of strict isolation (e.g. rabies). In some hospitals (e.g. in Asia) banana leaves may be used.

Mattresses and pillows

- Are a major source of cross-infection and contribute to bed sores.
- Soggy (wet) mattresses *must* be changed.
- Must be covered with an impervious layer so that they can be cleaned thoroughly between patients.
- Clean with warm water and detergent.
- Damaged and cotton-covered mattresses filled with horse-hair (or other fibres that can become contaminated) can be a source of cross-infection with spores, e.g. *Clostridium tetani*.
- Never admit new patients onto soiled, stained, or contaminated mattresses.

Rubber covers can be uncomfortable in hot countries. It may be possible to cover the mattress cover with absorbable paper, which should be changed frequently.

Thermometers

- Wash in warm water and detergent and dry.
- Wipe over with a swab or cotton wool ball soaked in 70 per cent isopropyl alcohol.
- Never soak in disinfectants.

Trolley tops

- Wipe with warm water and detergent to remove dust.
- Dry.

Nail brushes

- These are not recommended for ward use.
- Single-use disposable or autoclavable brushes should be used for specialized wards.

Glass ampoules

To avoid sharps injury, hold top with cotton wool or tissue paper before breaking open.

Specialized equipment

Endoscopy unit

Fibre optics

These are usually heat-labile and therefore require chemical disinfection:

- Use 2 per cent glutaraldehyde under strictly controlled conditions (see Health and Safety, p. 176).
- Ensure that the correct type of aldehyde (which does not damage the equipment) is used.

Procotoscopes and sigmoidoscopes

These can be disposable or reusable. Disposable ones may be more economical, as reusable ones must be cleaned, sterilized, or disinfected by heat or 2 per cent glutaraldehyde.

Intensive care unit, operating theatres, etc.
Ventilatory circuits

- Multiple-use circuits must be heat-disinfected for at least 80°C for 3 minutes or autoclaved (check manufacturer's guidelines) between each patient. Ethylene oxide is an alternative.
- The use of undisinfected circuits between patients increases the risk of chest infection due to Gram-negative bacilli, e.g. *Pseudomonas aeruginosa*.
- Shortage of equipment may necessitate the use of the same circuit up to 72 hours for the same patient. As long as the circuit has not been contaminated this is acceptable. Install filters on the expiratory and inspiratory ends of the ventilator to prevent contamination.
- Filters may be used between patients and ventilator circuits increase the usage time.
- If properly maintained, a ventilated patient may use the same circuit for 4–5 days before disinfection becomes necessary.
- Heat exchange filters (Pall filters) eliminate the need for humidifiers, but are expensive.

The pathogens that can survive in moisture and mucus are:

- bacterial pathogens:
  - —*Haemophilus influenzae*;
  - —*Streptococcus pneumoniae* and other streptococci;
  - —*Staphylococcus aureus*;
  - —Gram-negative bacilli, e.g. *Pseudomonas*;
- *Mycobacterium tuberculosis*;
- viral pathogens;
- *Mycoplasma pneumoniae*.

Humidifiers

These are a common source of Gram-negative bacilli (and viruses) associated with respiratory tract infection:

- empty daily;
- refill with sterile water;
- disinfect when contaminated—wash and leave in a solution of 1 per cent hypochlorite for 30 minutes then wash thoroughly and dry;

- routine heat disinfection is essential after each patient use;
- if humidification is required for a prolonged period the humidifier should be cleaned thoroughly, dried, and filled daily with sterile water;
- the humidifier should be heat-disinfected when the respiratory circuit is changed;
- humidifiers should never be topped up from the tap.

Alternatively: Respiratory microbial and humidifying filters fitted to the ventilator circuits act as a barrier and provide moisture from the patient's breath.

If SSD facilities are available, autoclavable circuits are most cost-effective but filters are more convenient.

Endotracheal suction catheters

- These are usually disposable but may be used for up to 24 hours on the same patient, provided that the catheter is stored properly and does not become contaminated.
- The water used for flushing the catheter after each suction must be sterile and changed every time.
- The bowl must be washed and dried after each suction and filled with sterile water only before use.

Alternatively:

- Where there is a shortage of supplies the catheters may be used for more than 24 hours (and possibly until the patient leaves the unit) provided that the catheter is stored properly and rinsed out thoroughly after each use.
- Nursing staff and attendants must disinfect their hands properly before and after each use.
- Suction catheters must not be shared between patients.

Endotracheal tubes

- These may be recycled after thorough cleaning and autoclaving.
- Disposable endotracheal tubes are available but are more expensive than recyclable ones.

- Reports of allergic reactions to the red rubber used in endo-tracheal tubes has led manufacturers to use equally heat-resistant but less reactive materials.

Ambu-bags

These are used for resuscitation and, in developing countries, relatives usually help ventilate the patient. Ambu-bags are extremely difficult to disinfect and become contaminated very quickly:

- Heat is the most reliable method of disinfection; 2 per cent glutaraldehyde is a less acceptable alternative.
- The bags must be rinsed thoroughly in sterile water after immersing in glutaraldehyde. This will reduce the risk of chemical irritation, which can itself precipitate respiratory infection.

Oxygen-delivery face masks

These can be disposable or reusable. If reused:

- Wash thoroughly.
- Dry and wipe over with 70 per cent isopropyl alcohol. This will remove mucus.

Suction and drainage bottles

- These are usually disposable, with a self-sealing inner container held in a clear plastic outer container.
- Before buying a system, ensure that the outer container can be heat-disinfected or autoclaved.

Non-disposable bottles:

- Must be changed every 24 hours (or sooner if full).
- The contents may be emptied down the sluice.
- Must be rinsed and sent to the SSD for autoclaving.
- If autoclaving facilities are not available, wash thoroughly and dry.
- Recyclable connector tubing should be cleaned thoroughly and sterilized. The system must be closed and risk to staff from body fluids should be minimal.
- Do not leave fluids standing in suction bottles.

Neonatal and paediatric units
Respiratory equipment
See Ventilator Circuits (p. 121).

Incubators
- Clean thoroughly with warm soapy water to remove organic contamination.
- Dry and wipe over with 70 per cent isopropyl alcohol.

Humidifiers
- Empty daily. Wash and dry.
- Refill with sterile water.
- Disinfect when contaminated—wash and leave in a solution of 1 per cent hypochlorite for 2 hours. Then wash thoroughly and dry.

Resuscitaires
- Disconnect all connections.
- Wash thoroughly with a soft brush.
- Send to SSD for autoclaving.

Disposable equipment
Needles and syringes
- These present a high risk of blood-borne disease (see p. 124).
- Fine-born needles cannot be cleaned and therefore should not be recycled.

Recycling of syringes must be well controlled. After thorough cleaning, the syringes must be autoclaved or processed in ethylene oxide.

Administration sets
- Administration sets for i.v. fluids must be disposable—they carry the same risks as cannulae.

Alternatively:
- Recycle but use for a completely different purpose, e.g. draining urinary catheters.

Urinary catheters and drainage bags

These should be single-use and disposable (see Urinary Catheterization Policy, p. 51).

Alternative use of equipment for countries with minimal resources

Disinfection and sterilization

Boiling invasive instruments, e.g. glass syringes and metal catheters, on the wards is hazardous and should be discouraged. The SSD has facilities to cater for all ward equipment and sterilizes much more efficiently and safely. This also takes pressure off the already over-worked nursing staff.

Boiling pasteurizers

- The temperature is often poorly controlled and the presence of steam or boiling water does not necessarily mean that 100 °C has been reached.

- The deposit of calcium around the inner chamber may harbour bacteria, viruses, and spores that are not killed by the lower-than-optimal temperatures achieved.

- Equipment (and small-bore items in particular, e.g. needles and urinary catheters) cannot be cleaned adequately and is therefore inadequately penetrated by heat.

- Equipment from different patients is mixed in the same cycle and, if there is inadequate sterilization, cross-infection can occur.

All surgical instruments must be autoclaved under properly controlled conditions.
Soaking equipment in disinfectants is unreliable.

Pressure cookers

In remote areas, basic amenities such as electricity or gas are not available. Here pressure cookers, with a reinforced gasket, may be used to sterilize solid metal surgical instruments. The cookers reach 121 °C at 103.5 kPa but there is no vacuum to allow steam penetration, so hollow-bore instruments cannot be sterilized reliably.

Items of disposable equipment are often used for purposes other than those for which they were intended. Ingenious ways of using such equipment keep costs down and fulfil some of the needs of the patients. Provided that the principles of infection control are maintained these are acceptable as interim measures.

Administration sets

These can be used for:

- Urinary drainage into i.v. bottles, either for connecting a urinary catheter to a drainage bag or for connecting an i.v. fluid bottle for urinary drainage:
  —the system must fit snugly;
  —a closed circuit must be maintained;
  —there must be no leakage of urine.
  —it is best to recycle the administration set and bottle to the same patient.
- Distributing air to neonates from a communal tank of oxygen, although it is difficult to understand how oxygen can flow through such a narrow tube, especially when a hypodermic needle is used to link into the other sets for channelling oxygen. A better alternative might be larger bore suction tubes with a three-way valve connector.

Urinary catheters

In countries that experience difficulties in supply or funding, patients may be expected to buy their own urinary catheters, or the hospital may provide recycled catheters for them. Recommendations are:

- Buy two urinary catheters for long-term patients, e.g. those with neurogenic bladders. These should be clearly labelled with the patient's name or identification number, and should be recycled only to that patient. This is not entirely satisfactory, but it is better than using someone else's catheter.
- Disinfect recycled urinary catheters by autoclaving (preferable) or with 2 per cent glutaraldehyde and at least four to five rinses with sterile water. If catheters are often not properly flushed-through after disinfection some glutaraldehyde may be retained and this can lead to urethral strictures.

I.v. fluid bottles

These have been used for:

- urinary drainage;
- chest drain;
- suction.

Provided that a closed circuit is maintained, with well fitting connections, and the equipment is not constantly dismantled to be emptied, it should be acceptable.

Oxygen delivery masks for neonates

Paper cones with a rubber tube attachment to provide oxygen for the babies are acceptable provided that a separate mask and tube is used for each neonate.

Hot water bottles

When baby incubators are not available, hot water bottles covered with several layers of cloth (to prevent burning or scalding) are quite acceptable.

Alternatively: Use an angle-poise table lamp with a large bulb.

Latex gloves

These can be cut into strips and sterilized for use as intra-abdominal drains. Pieces of administration set are also used but neither is recommended.

Cleaning patient-care equipment

Clean with warm water and detergent—low risk

- patients' personal articles;
- crockery and cutlery, glasses, and jugs;
- mattresses and pillow cases;
- wash basins and similar equipment.
- floors and walls.

Heat disinfection—medium risk

- bedpans, urinals, and urine jugs;

- Cheatle forceps—store dry;
- floor mops;
- suction bottles (if heat-sensitive these can be disinfected at < 80 °C).

Autoclaving—high risk

- all surgical instruments;
- dressings;
- recycled syringes, etc.

Table 7.1 shows alternative methods to autoclaving as a first choice.

Table 7.1 Alternatives to autoclaving

Equipment	Alternative methods
Suction bottles, drainage bottles for wounds, etc.	Use disposable items Wash and dry then wipe with hypochlorite
Oxygen tubing and suction tubing	Treat with glutaraldehyde for 30 min RINSE THOROUGHLY BEFORE USE
Forceps (Cheatle)	Wash and dry thoroughly Wipe over with 70 % isopropyl alcohol
Surgical instruments	No alternative
Wound dressings	No alternative
Paediatric equipment	
bottles and teats (keep separate for each baby)	Boil for 10 min and then dry OR Store in Milton liquid
humidifier	Wash and dry. Fill with 1 % hypochlorite and leave for 2 hours. Wash thoroughly and dry MUST BE HEAT STERILIZED IF TO BE USED FOR VENTILATION
ventilator circuits	Use disposable items 2 % glutaraldehyde
incubator	Wipe and dry. Wipe with 70 % isopropyl alcohol CANNOT BE HEAT DISINFECTED

Intensive therapy unit

The Intensive Therapy Unit (ITU) is one of the busiest units in the hospital and uses some of the most sophisticated equipment and advanced medical practices. However, the ITU contributes to more nosocomial and cross-infections that other wards. Although infections arising in ITU patients may be endogenous, as the patients require high dependency nursing, there is more potential for considerable cross-infection from the hands of staff and from equipment. Policies for the ITU must be clear and must be meticulously implemented.

Main areas of cross-infection in the ITU

- hands of staff and attendants (via two-bowl hand-washing and communal towels);
- assisted ventilation equipment;
- suction and drainage bottles;
- i.v. lines—central and peripheral;
- urinary catheters;
- wounds and wound dressings;
- disinfectant containers;
- dressing trolleys (on which disinfectnt jars/bottles are stored).

Policies relating to infection control

These should include:

- *Layout of unit and siting of equipment.* The unit should ideally be situated close to the operating theatre and Accident and Emergency Department and should be readily accessible, but separate, from the main ward areas. The unit usually contains six to ten beds, including one or two isolation cubicles for communicable diseases. The beds should be 2.5–3 metres (7–9 feet) apart, to allow free movement of staff and equipment. The ITU should function independently, with a dedicated nursing staff who are well-trained in the management of high dependency patients and are familiar with infection control principles.

- *Admissions policy.* Any patient with diarrhoea, excoriating skin conditions or a recognized communicable disease, or who is a known carrier of an epidemic strain of bacterium, should be admitted directly to an isolation cubicle with dedicated equipment and staff. He/she may be moved out to the open ward once they have cleared by the clinical microbiologist or IC team.

- *Disinfection and sterilization of specialized equipment.* This should not be carried in the ITU—all equipment should be sent to the SSD. A policy on disposable and reusable items should be clearly defined.

- *Hand disinfection.* (see Hand Disinfection Policy, p. 44). Hands are the most common vehicle of transmission of organisms and so facilities should be provided for hand washing and disinfection. A container of alcohol—chlorhexidine (Hibisol) should be available at the entrance (where the white coats are removed), opposite the nursing station and next to each end. Wash-hand basins must be provided. All visitors and staff should decontaminate their hands before touching any patient. Preferably, each patient should have his/her dedicated Hibisol container next to their bed.

- *Aseptic procedures for intravenous therapy and urinary catheterization.* See Chapter 5, p. 42.

- *Protective clothing:*
  —gloves (sterile for aseptic procedures, e.g. insertion of CVP lines and non-sterile for other procedures, e.g. emptying urinary drainage bags);
  —plastic aprons when dealing with patient body fluids;
  —overshoes and headgear are not required;
  —disposable high-efficiency filter masks for aseptic procedures.

- *Antibiotic and disinfectant usage:*
  —this must be restricted to essential use only. An antibiotic policy on prophylaxis and empirical therapy is essential and should be prescribed with logic and restraint;
  —selective gut decontamination by non-antimicrobials should be considered for reducing endogenous infection;
  —emergence of antibiotic resistance amongst bacteria;
  —disinfectants should be kept to a minimum and should never

be stored in open containers. Wherever possible, heat disinfection should be used;

—all equipment should be sent to the SSD to be sterilized.

- *Cleaning programme*:
  —cleaning must be done daily and all surfaces must be wiped with a damp cloth to remove dust and dirt;
  —disinfectants are not required for environmental cleaning (unless specified, e.g. for an unusual outbreak);
  —the main ward should be cleaned first and then the cubicles;
  —a total clean of all areas, including the stores, should be done at least every 2 weeks.
  —all equipment should be wiped and kept covered to protect from dust when not in use.

- *Visitors (including staff) to the ITU* should follow the same protocol:
  —street coats and white coats must be removed;
  —hands should be disinfected with alcohol—chlorhexidine (Hibisol) on entering the ITU;
  —the proper procedure should be followed when attending the patient;
  —hands should be disinfected before leaving the unit.

- *Waste and sharps disposal* (see pp. 33–42):
  —there must be adequate facilities for disposing of body fluids, excrement, clinical and non-clinical waste;
  —a sharps policy must be implemented and followed. The ITU is a busy area and there is a high risk from inoculation accidents. This could be one of the areas where self-resheathing needles and cannulae (see p. 96) could be used, although these are cumbersome to use and expensive.

- *Staff*:
  —there must be adequate work and rest facilities;
  —all staff working on the unit must be offered hepatitis B immunization;
  —training and education should consist of formal and informal infection control lectures and tutorial, and ward rounds.

The IC team should visit the ITU regularly. The IC doctor can advise on medical matters, while the IC nurse can advise on aseptic procedures.

Cost-saving alternatives in the ITU are highlighted in Table 7.2.

Table 7.2 ITU equipment and alternatives for reducing cost

Item	First choice	Second choice
Gloves: sterile	Disposable	Fresh pair
non-sterile	Disposable	Recycled
Aprons, plastic	Disposable	Recycled—wipe with alcohol. Dedicated to each patient
Mask—high efficiency filter	Disposable	No alternative
Ventilator tubing	Protective filters	Heat disinfected 2 % glutaraldehyde
Ventilator machines	Protection filters	Hydrogen peroxide internal clean
I.v. cannula	Disposable, change within 72 hours	No alternative
CV lines	Disposable, change if infected or as necessary	No alternative
Administration sets	Disposable, change every 48–72 hours	Change as necessary
Urinary catheters	Disposable	Recycle with heat disinfection, ethylene oxide, and recycle to same patient
Catheter bags	Disposable after each patient	Empty ? heat disinfection
Wound dressing	Sterile, disposable	No alternative
Endotracheal suction catheter	Disposable	Use for same patient then discard
Suction bottles	Disposable Autoclave	Heat sterilized

Operating theatres

Infection control in the operating theatre has been the subject of considerable discussion. Vast improvements have been made to the air supply, theatre procedure, surgical technique, and antibiotic prophylaxis, It is now accepted that good surgical technique and practice plays an important part in prevention of post-operative wound infection, provided that satisfactory theatre facilities are made available.

Generally, the operating theatre should have a clean environment with sufficient air changes to reduce the counts (at the wound site) of bacteria dispersed by personnel during an operation. However, for implant surgery, the environment should be ultra-clean, with minimal bacterial contamination from the air and personnel. Whether the theatres are for general or dedicated use, the principles are the same. It is sensible, but not essential, to organize the operating lists so that the clean cases are at the beginning of the list.

Points to consider

Siting of the operating theatre suites

Operating theatres may be sited in either purpose-built units or converted hospital accommodation. They are busy units and therefore require considerable planning and discussion before they are built, to prevent expensive mistakes. They should be sited within easy reach of the surgical wards and the Accident and Emergency Department to facilitate easy access for the patients. They should be separated from the main flow of hospital traffic and from the main corridors. The floor should be coved, with antistatic material, and the walls should be painted with impervious, antistatic paint; this reduces the dust levels and allows frequent cleaning. The surfaces should withstand frequent cleaning and hypochlorite decontamination.

Layout of the operating theatre

The operating theatre should be zoned (Table 7.3), and aseptic and clean areas should be separated from the outer areas. This is easier to achieve in purpose-built units and physical barriers may be needed in converted theatre units to restrict access and maintain unidirectional movement.

No-one should enter the theatre complex without changing into a fresh theatre suit.

The outer zone

This should contain:

- a main access corridor;
- accessible area for the removal of waste;

Table 7.3 A suggested layout for an operating theatre complex

Zone	Barrier	Areas included
Dirty/outside	Physical	Sluice, storage, waste disposal, outside corridor, changing rooms
Clean	Partial	Supply store, disinfection room, anaesthetic room, recovery room
Aseptic	Operating room	Sterile preparation, autoclave access

- a sluice;
- storage for medical and surgical supplies;
- an entrance to the changing facilities.

There is no need to change into theatre clothes to enter these areas but further acccess to the operating suite should be restricted..

The clean zone
This contains:

- the sterile supplies store;
- an anaesthetic room;
- a recovery area;
- scrub-up area;
- a clean corridor;
- rest rooms for staff.

Entry to this areas needs a change into theatre clothes and shoes, but there is no need for mask, gloves, or gown. There should be unidirectional access from this area to the aseptic area, preferable via the scrub-up area. The staff may not always need to scrub up before entering the operating room, and access to the operating area is therefore restricted. If the staff have to leave, they should do so via the changing area.

Aseptic area
This area should be restricted to the working team. It includes:

- the operating room;
- sterile preparation room.

Staff working in this area should change into theatre clothes, wear masks and gowns and, where necessary, sterile gloves.

Temperature and humidity

The temperature (72 °C) and humidity (not less than 55 per cent) play a very important role in maintaining staff and patient comfort. They must be carefully regulated and monitored. In low humidity, there is a danger of electrostatic sparks.

Ideally, the operating room should be 1 °C cooler than the outer area. This aids the outward movement of air, with the warmer air rising and cooler air moving to replace it.

Air supply

The air supply to each operating theatre suite should be independent, so that it can be switched off and maintained without affecting the entire theatre complex. If this is not feasible, each unit should supply no more than two separate suites.

Air is supplied to the operating theatre by:

Plenum ventilation

This is the most frequently used system in general purpose operating rooms:

- Atmospheric air is filtered and delivered to the operating room and sterile preparation area via ducts in the ceiling.
- A coarse filter to remove dust and debris is installed after the atmospheric air has been drawn into the air handling unit (AHU).
- A bacterial filter (2 μm or less with 95 per cent efficiency) is placed just inside the inlet grill.
- The air should be propelled through the ducts by a fan calculated to deliver 20–24 air changes per hour (1000–15 000 cubic feet per minute to the operating room), depending on the volume of air in the room.
- The air is partially extracted via ducts in the ceiling and partially via unidirectional baffle plate outlets in the doors, to ensure adequate circulation. Some air is recirculated within the suite.
- An exhaust system in the corridors and the sluice room then removes the air to the atmosphere outside.

- The bacterial counts at the wound site should be no more than 100–500 bacteria-carrying particles (BCP) per cubic metre.

Laminar flow ventilation (ultra clean ventilation)

This system is unidirectional and delivers air flows over the operating table of 300 air changes per hour and a bacterial count of 10 BCP or less per cubic metre at the wound site:

- Air is drawn in from the atmosphere and passes through a 5 μm filter to 95 per cent efficiency.

- Approximately 80 per cent of the air in the room is recycled through a canopy over the operating table and passes through a 5 μm filter.

- Before the air is delivered to the operating site it passes through a high efficiency particulate air (HEPA) filter with a 0.3 μm filter and 99.97 per cent efficiency, which removes bacterial contamination.

Laminar flow ventilation is very expensive and is usually used in specialized orthopaedic units, often in conjunction with sophisticated close surgical suites. Laminar flow may be delivered vertically or horizontally; the former is preferable. Regular service and maintenance of the ventilation plant is essential. This is usually carried out annually but may require more frequent cleaning in countries with high atmospheric dust and pollution.

There should not be reversal of air flows when exits are opened nor any leakage through the seals around the doors and windows when they are closed.

Wall-mounted air conditioners

These are installed in some tropical countries, more for comfort than for clean air delivery; they should not be used as air delivery systems. The units are usually mounted on the outside wall, which is hot, and the air is directed down and back onto itself towards the wall. The operating table does not receive any significant air changes and the bacterial counts remain unaffected.

Free-standing air conditioners

These are cooling units, with no filtration of air, and therefore do not fulfil the criteria for air delivery systems.

Staff

There is a well-documented correlation between the number of people in the operating suite and an increase in bacterial counts. It is estimated that each person in the suite creates 10 000 viable organisms per minute when at rest, increasing to 50 000 when moving. There should therefore be only essential staff in the operating suite and they should not move more than is necessary. Opening and closing of the outer doors should be kept to a minimum.

Equipment

Equipment such as suction apparatus and ventilators must be fitted with bacterial filters to prevent contamination of the machines (see Specialized Equipment, p. 121). All the dirty instruments should be counted, carefully rinsed to remove superficial contamination, if the policy requires, and sent to the TSSU for sterilization. If a known case of HIV or hepatitis B is involved, the instruments should be clearly labelled and sent directly to TSSU with minimal handling.

Waste

- Waste should be disposed of with minimal handling because there is a risk of hepatitis B and HIV transmission.
- Body fluids can be disposed of in the sluice with appropriate protective clothing, such as gloves, aprons, and eye protection.
- Equipment should not be rinsed before sending to the TSSU and it should be clearly labelled if it is from a high-risk patient.
- Dirty linen should be taken to the sluice, bagged in a colour-coded bag and labelled.
- All waste requiring incineration should be placed into water-proof bags and marked for incineration.

Cleaning programme

There should be a simple, clear policy that can be adhered to easily. The cleaning equipment for the operating room must be dedicated and kept separate from the outer zone.

Spillage of blood and body fluids

(See p. 95.) This is the only indication for use of an environmental disinfectant for spot cleaning in the operating theatre.

Daily cleaning

This should be carried out after the operating sessions are over:

- All the surfaces should be cleaned with detergent and water dried.
- Wipe walls to head height (2.5–3 metres) every day.
- Scrub floors with warm water and detergent and dry. No disinfectant in necessary.
- Wipe operating table and other non-clinical equipment to remove all visible dirt and leave to dry.
- Clean sluice with warm water and detergent.
- Wipe over non-metallic surfaces and equipment to remove contamination.
- Clean slop-hopper, non-clinical equipment, and containers.

Weekly cleaning

- Clean all the areas inside the operating theatre complex with warm water and detergent. Dry.
- Empty storage shelves, wipe over, dry, and restack.

Ultraviolet sterilization of the theatre suites is expensive, ineffective, and an unnecessary waste of resources.

Maintenance

- Equipment should be checked every week (or fortnightly at the most).
- Ventilation must be checked monthly and the filters changed as required (usually annually).

The IC team should be told whenever the air delivery system has been worked on, so that the bacterial counts and the air flows can be checked in conjunction with the engineers. The theatre should be used only after clearance from the IC team.

It is advisable to have back-up theatre facilities so that theatre sessions are not interrupted by maintenance.

Other points to consider

- suction;
- piped gas;

- water supply;
- storage;
- changing areas;
- anaesthetic rooms;
- recovery area;
- scrub-up area;
- sterile preparation area;
- sterile services for dressings, packs, sterile gowns, and surgical instruments;
- health and morale of staff working in the unit.

Commissioning operating theatres

The IC team should be involved in any planning and commissioning of operating theatres, in conjunction with the engineers and architects. It is advisable for the IC team to visit the building site during construction to ensure that the layout, ventilation system, and facilities comply with the specifications.

Testing the new theatres should be done on a specified date after they have been cleaned and are ready for use, but before they are operational. The bacteriology results take at least 48 hours and the theatres should not be used until the tests are complete. An annual record of the air flows and bacterial counts for each operating theatre should be kept. This is useful as a comparison in the future.

Bacterial counts

These are done with an air-sampling device—either a Casella slit sampler or a Biotest air sampler:

- *Casella slit sampler.* This is a large vacuum extractor with a nozzle, which is pointed towards the area to be sampled. A known quantity or air (between 30 and 70 litres per minute) is passed directly over an agar plate for a given time (usually 4 or 8 minutes). The plate is then incubated and the number of BCPs are calculated per cubic metre of air. Acceptable levels are 100–500 BCP per cubic metre for conventionally ventilated operating theatres and 10 BCP per cubic metre for ultra-clean ventilation. There should be no more than one colony of *Clostridium perfringens* or *Staphylococcus aureus* per plate.

- *Biotest sampler.* This is smaller than the slit sampler and is portable, with a centrifugal fan that draws air in and passes it over a strip of agar, which is placed facing the air.

Although the Biotest sampler is more convenient, all the calculations for laminar flow systems have been made on the slit sampler, which is now the standard. A template should be made of the different areas to be sampled, starting from the air inlet and the operating table and working outwards to the exits. Rooms that lead off the operating room, including the sluice, should also be sampled. The same template can be used for subsequent tests.

Bacterial counts are also useful when investigating an outbreak where the operating theatre environment may be in question or where a member of the theatre staff may be a suspected disperser of the outbreak strain.

NOTE. It is important that the person carrying out the tests is not a 'shedder', as this will effect the results and give a false reading.

Settle plates

These are not used routinely because bacterial counts in air cannot be calculated accurately and reflect only the presence of bacteria, which in itself is meaningless, unless a know pathogen is being investigated.

Air flows

Air flows are examined using an innocuous smoke-producing substance, such as titanium chloride:

- A swab or 'smoke bomb' is held under the inlet grill and the air movements are followed around the operating theatre and out through the doors.
- The floor seals and baffle outlets should be checked.
- The air flows are then followed to the outer zone and to the extract ventilators and grills.
- Any reversal of air flow, particularly from the outer zone inwards, should be recorded and corrected.

Air changes

The engineers should perform tests to check that new filters have not decreased the air changes. Any alteration should be corrected immediately.

Theatre sterile services unit (TSSU)

- The TSSU is usually under the control of the operating theatre manager but may be incorporated into a larger central unit. In some units all the sterilization takes place within the theatre complex.

- The supply of surgical instruments should be sufficient to maintain an adequate supply for concurrent operations and sterilization.

- On-site sterilization is feasible only if the TSSU possesses autoclaves and if there are proper facilities for washing and processing contaminated instruments. To ensure proper quality control, it may be more sensible to centralize the service.

- If TSSU services are available, the only facilities needed in the operating theatre are for rapid sterilization of dropped instrument (134 °C for 3.5 minutes) and to decontaminate fibre optics. The latter must be carried out in well-controlled conditions (see below).

Disinfectants

(See Health and Safety, p. 172). There is little need for disinfectants in an operating theatre, apart from skin disinfection for the patient and hands of the staff, and after spillage of blood and body fluids.

Heat-labile equipment

2 per cent glutaraldehyde can be used for heat-labile equipment, e.g. endoscopes and gastroscopes, although its use must be carefully controlled. Glutaraldehyde should always be used with adequate ventilation or in an exhaust cabinet, and a closed system for washing and soaking the fibre optics is recommended, with at least three rinses in sterile water to remove all traces of the disinfectant.

Skin disinfection

(See Disinfection, p. 44.):

- The patient's skin should be prepared with 40 per cent isopropyl alcohol (NOTE: the usual concentration of 70 per cent isopropyl alcohol has been reduced because of the danger of ignition and burns from diathermy). This is usually combined with a sustained-action disinfectant, e.g. chlorhexidine or povidone iodine (povidone iodine may be preferred for implant surgery, as it reduces the bacterial and spore counts, but chlorhexidine is equally effective).

- Some surgeons advocate total body washing with chlorhexidine prior to operation. This is a matter of personal choice.

Surgical hand washing

- A 2-minute scrub with a sustained-action disinfectant, such as chlorhexidine or povidone iodine is recommended. Recent evidence suggests that scrubbing with a brush is no longer recommended.
- Further scrubbing is not necessary but there should be a 2-minute wash with the disinfectants mentioned above. The initial scrub removes all dust and grime, further scrubbing can damage the skin and increase bacterial colonization.
- The scrubbing brush, if used, should be single-use only and should be autoclaved or discarded. Brushes must *not* be left soaking in a open disinfectant bowl—this can result in colonization with Gram-negative bacilli (see Hand Disinfection, p. 44).

Shaving patient operation sites

This has been very controversial and is subject to changing fashions and practices.

- It is now recommended that only the incision area is cleared of hair in the anaesthetic room.
- The patient's skin should not be traumatized, as this may increase wound infection rates.
- Depilatory creams are no longer recommended because of possible damage to the patient's skin.

The arguments about shaving continue.

Protective clothing for use in the operating theatre
Gowns

- Cotton gowns have a pore size of 80–100 μm and allow the passage of skin organisms.

- GoreTex gowns are made of PTFE film laminated to one or two layers of woven fabric, e.g. polyester, and have a pore diameter of 0.2 μm.
- A cheaper alternative is tightly woven washable fabric such as polycotton.

The most recent recommendations are that gowns should be made of non-woven bio-occlusive material—not cotton. This reduces the bacterial contamination from the surgeon to the patient. In ortho-paedics, closed systems are considered more appropriate, although these are uncomfortable and difficult to work in for long periods of time.

In known cases of HIV of hepatitis B, a plastic apron under the gown is recommended, to reduce contamination from blood.

Masks

Only high efficiency filter masks are recommended and must be changed after each operation. These are now considered to be worn mainly for protection for the operators from splash contamination rather than as a bacterial barrier. Cotton masks are not considered protective in either situation.

Gloves

Well fitting latex sterile surgical gloves are worn by all operators. Where the HIV or hepatitis B status of the patient is known (i.e. is positive) double gloving is now recommended. Although this is more cumbersome to work with, it offers more protection to needle-stick injuries than single gloves.

Boots/shoes

The recent recommendations are a change of footwear whilst in theatre. Surgeons dealing with heavy blood or body fluid con-tamination are advised to wear boots that are adequately covered by the plastic apron to avoid fluid from going into the shoes/boots.

Headgear

The hair must be covered completely, whether by disposable or recyclable coverings. In hot countries, headgear should be changed frequently.

Staff health

- No member of staff with open skin lesions should handle patients
- No surgeon should operate with uncovered cuts and abrasions—all cuts and abrasions must be covered with a water-proof dressing.
- Staff with coughs and colds should not be allowed into the operating area, although they may work in the outer zone.
- All staff must be offered hepatitis B immunization.
- Morale. Theatre staff work intensively for long hours and morale is very important. Adequate rest facilities must be provided inside the theatre complex so that staff do not need to change in and out of their theatre clothes. There should be somewhere to relax and take refreshments.

Summary

- Air should flow from the central operating area outwards to the clean zone and then to the outer zone.
- *Patient movement*: enter theatre complex; transfer on to internal trolley; enter clean corridor; enter anaesthetic room; enter operating theatre; exit operating theatre via recovery room.
- *Staff movement*: enter changing rooms; enter clean area; enter operating theatre (or where required); enter rest rooms; exit via changing rooms.
- *Instruments*: used instruments to dirty sluice and then to SSD, where they are washed, processed, packed, sterilized, and returned to the sterile store in the operating suite.

Burns unit

This is a highly specialized unit that, given the nature of the patient admitted, lends itself to colonization and infection with organisms that are difficult to treat. The patent's defences are lowered and direct contact with staff and equipment is high.

Again, hands are the most important source of cross-infection, followed by environmental factors, such as air-borne skin scales.

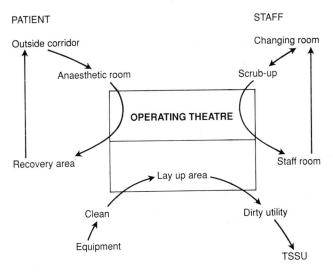

Fig. 7.1 Movement of theatre staff, patients, and equipment into the operating theatre.

Design and layout

The burns unit should:

- be purpose-built and self-contained, with a number of single-use cubicles;
- have an independent ventilation system;
- not be sited near areas that may contribute to environmental contamination.

Nosocomial organisms frequently found in the burns unit

- *Staphylococcus aureus* (MRSA);
- Group A streptococci;
- Gram-negative bacilli (multiply antibiotic-resistant);
- *Pseudomonas aeruginosa*;
- *Acinetobacter* species;
- *Enterobacter* species;
- *Klebsiella* species;
- *Aspergillus* species;

- *Candida* species;
- Fungi.

Points to consider

- The unit must be dedicated to burns patients.
- The unit should be separate from the main ward and busy hospital areas.
- The air introduced to the unit must be clean and filtered for dust and bacteria before delivery (See Plenum Ventilation, p. 135).
- The air may be supplied:
  —from an air-handling unit and delivered via separate ducts to each cubicle; *or*
  —to a central lobby and then to the rooms.
  The former is more desirable.
- Single cubicles must be provided with air extraction to the outside atmosphere and minimal recycling of air should be permitted.
- If possible, separate operating theatre facilities should be provided. If this is not possible, burns patients should be dealt with in a separate session in the general operating theatre—the clean patients should be seen before the dirty cases.

Despite all precautions, colonization is high and the extensive use of antibiotics and topical products adds to an increase in multiply antibiotic-resistant Gram-negative bacilli.

Policies

Policies for the burns unit should include:

- Complete change of clothing for full-time staff.
- Sterile gowns, gloves, and masks for visitors; overshoes are not necessary.
- Hand washing facilities must be readily available. Alcohol—chlorhexidine should be put next to each bed to be used by all staff before and after contact with patients or equipment.
- Aseptic procedures (see p. 42).
- Disposable urinary catheters should be used, recycled catheters are not recommended.

- Water-proof mattresses, which can be washed and dried regularly and wiped over with a disinfectant (hypochlorite) if necessary.

- Sterile clinical equipment and disinfected non-clinical equipment should be properly tested and subject to quality control.

- Linen must be disinfected but, where patients are treated by exposure, sterile linen is indicated and needs to be changed daily.

- Dedicated equipment should be used for each patient. Where there is a shortage of ventilator tubing, bedpans, etc. and equipment has be shared, a clear policy on sterilization and disinfection is necessary.

- There should be a regular and frequent cleaning programme:
  —the floors, walls, and ceiling should be cleaned with warm water and detergent.
  —each room should be cleaned thoroughly after the patient has left and should be allowed to dry before admitting further patients.

- Waste disposal should be carried out safely and effectively according to the colour-coding policy (see p. 40).

- Staff must be highly trained and understand the principles of infection control. They should be provided with satisfactory rest facilities.

- All staff should be offered hepatitis B immunization.

The IC team should visit the burns regularly and help in the formulation of unit policies and ensure that supplies of essential sterile and non-sterile equipment are available. They should always be available to advise on matters relating to infection control.

Summary

- The burns unit should be independent of the rest of the hospital, with isolation cubicles and ventilation
- It should have well-thought-out policies on:
  —hand washing;
  —disinfection and sterilization;
  —antibiotic policies;
  —cleaning and waste disposal.

Bone marrow transplant unit

Many countries are embarking on bone marrow transplant programmes. The bone marrow transplant unit is a high dependency nursing unit where the patients are immunosuppressed over a long period of time and are therefore prone to bacterial, viral, and fungal infections from exogenous and endogenous sources.

Points to consider
Design and layout of the unit
- The unit should be purpose-built and must be well away from possible sources of contamination, particularly fungal spores.
- The doors and windows should be well-sealed.
- The unit should be divided into single rooms with integrated toilet and washing facilities. Each room should have at least one anteroom for storage of patient care articles, food, and protective clothing for the staff and visitors. Hand-washing facilities must be provided in this area.
- There should be easy access to all the facilities in the unit with entry into the patients' cubicles.
- Clinical equipment should be kept inside the cubicle.
- Facilities for pharmacy preparation should be available, preferably in laminar flow cabinets.
- There must be adequate staff facilities.

Laminar air flow systems
- Air flow ducts should be short and come directly off the air conditioning plant.
- Dedicated air conditioning is very expensive, having two ducts off one plant is acceptable.
- There should be two coarse filters removing 7 μm particles (dust, etc.) One filter should be placed immediately after the air conditioning unit and the other between the HEPA filter and the first coarse filter.
- HEPA filters capable of excluding >99.97 per cent of 0.3 μm particles and of producing a unidirectional laminar flow at an air speed of 9–27 metres per minute (approximately 30 air changes).

- The HEPA filters should be placed just above the room grill at the inlet.
- Coarse filters should be changed every 3–4 months, depending on the climatic conditions.
- HEPA filters should be changed every 6 months, or after air conditioning plant maintenance has been carried out.
- Microbiological environmental monitoring should follow (see p. 139).

Sterilization and disinfection

- Hands must be disinfected and dried properly. Hand decontamination facilities, e.g. a wash-hand basin and an alcoholic rub, should be available.
- Sterile disposable body coverings (gowns, etc.) gloves, and masks should be provided. Headgear depends on departmental policy.
- All equipment must be heat-sterilized or disposable.
- All articles for entertainment should be disinfected regularly (or sterilized with ethylene oxide).

Cleaning

- All areas must be cleaned daily using a dedicated, clean, damp cloth, which may be kept in the anteroom and should be discarded after each patient.
- Disinfection is not necessary.
- Toilets must be cleaned and wiped with bleach.
- Domestic staff must change clothes and wear protective clothing when entering the unit.

Back-up services

- The hospital engineer must be familiar with the air delivery units and other equipment. Maintenance and service contracts and regular maintenance of the HEPA filters are essential.
- Sterile services must be of a very high standard.
- Infection control advice must be available at all times.

Food preparation

- During the period of total neutropenia, the patient may be fed canned food, heated up in a microwave.

- Later, cooked food should be prepared with sterile water and meticulous cleanliness, with special attention to crockery and cutlery.
- Drinking water should be sterile or bottled (depending on availability).
- Fresh fruit and fruit salads are not allowed unless the fruit is peeled.
- All milk and dairy products must be sterilized.

Pharmaceutical products

- All drugs and intravenous therapy must be prepared in a laminar flow cabinet.
- The person handling the products must change into sterile protective clothing.
- All delivery systems should be sterile—recycling is not allowed.
- Left-over products should be discarded.

Microbiology specimens

- Patients should be screened weekly for bacterial pathogens, antibiotic-resistant bacteria, fungi, and viruses.
- The sites to be screened are: the nose, throat, perineal swab, hair, urine, and faeces.
- Environmental monitoring does not necessarily have to be done routinely, but may be required when ventilation systems are overhauled or when there is an outbreak.
- If infection is clinically noted, a total infective screen, including blood cultures (three) and blood for serology, should be investigated (see Microbiology investigations, p. 81).

Visitors

Visitors should follow the same precautions as the staff.

Education

Education of all visitors and staff, including porters and domestics, is essential to prevent infection in the burns unit.

Staff

- The staff should be dedicated and highly trained.
- All staff should be immunized against Rubella, hepatitis B, etc.
- No member of staff should report for duty with a cough, cold, flu-like illness, skin condition, or any communicable disease.
- All contact with communicable diseases must be reported to the nurse-in-charge.

8. *Other departments*

Hotel management

Domestic and portering department

The IC team should be involved with the tender for contracts for domestic and associated services, advising on:

- general cleaning schedules;
- terminal cleaning requirements;
- high-risk or dependency area cleaning;
- cleaning of the bedpan disinfector;
- cleaning schedules for dirty areas;
- cleaning the wash-hand dispensers and replacing stocks on the wards;
- damp dusting schedules;
- the use of disinfectants.

Hotel services

The Hotel Services Department is responsible for the standard of general cleanliness and for implementation of specific protocols, including the replacement of all toiletries and paper products.

Domestic services

Implementation of the colour-coding system is the responsibility of the domestic manager. In most hospitals, the ward domestic staff wash and dry the crockery and cutlery and are responsible for ward kitchens.

Education and training

The domestic staff should be education and trained in infection control policy by the IC team. Training should cover:

- protective clothing;
- how to manage isolation categories;

- transport of patients;
- cleaning-up spillages.

During such training periods the IC team may learn about incorrect practices that are being carried out in the hospital, and can advise the domestic staff on the correct procedure.

Catering, kitchens, and food preparation

Kitchens and food preparation areas are potential sources of food poisoning, so kitchen practices are very important. In the UK, the Food Act (1984), which was amended in 1986 under the National Health Service (Amendment) Act, focused on safe catering practices and health authorities are now held responsible for ensuring that catering practices are safe.

Safe code of practice

The IC team, in conjunction with the catering manager, should draw up codes of practice relating to:

- safe preparation and handling of food;
- food hygiene—reducing the risk of food poisoning and serving palatable and nutritious food;
- correct times and temperatures for cooking and storage;
- cleaning programmes for all areas and equipment;
- records of incidences of food poisoning;
- pre-employment screening of staff;
- staff health;
- personal hygiene and staff clothing.

Design and layout of hospital kitchens

Accommodation

- The kitchens should be separate from the main hospital area and should be easily accessible from the road, for ease of delivery.
- The kitchens should have separate areas for the reception of raw products and the preparation of cooked and uncooked food.

- There should be adequate storage facilities, at the right temperatures, for uncooked and raw foods (see below).
- Kitchen utensils should be dismantled and cleaned every day.
- There should plenty of hot water to wash utensils, serving equipment, and crockery.
- Adequate wash-hand facilities and toilet facilities for the staff must be provided.
- Adequate rest areas should be provided.

Food preparation
- Cooked and uncooked food should be dealt with in separate areas.
- The separate areas should be colour coded and contain dedicated utensils.
- Storage areas in the refrigerator should be defined and separate.
- The freezer should be compartmentalized.

If separate storage facilities are unavoidable, all food should be covered properly and particular care should be taken to avoid storing prepared food under meat (which might drip blood/juices).

Food separation
- Any food capable of supporting bacterial growth should be stored at below 6 °C (± 2 °C) or above 65 °C.
- Utensils should be washed at at least 60 °C, and an ideal temperature of 80 °C is recommended.
- All utensils and crockery must be dried thoroughly.
- Food should not be left unrefrigerated for over 2 hours.
- All foods should be stored appropriately on receipt.

Temperatures
Food storage
- Frozen foods should be transported and stored at temperatures of −13 to −18 °C.
- Cold foods should be transported and stored at no more than 5 °C.

- Freezers should be kept at at least −18 °C and fridges at no higher than 4 °C.

Food preparation
- Meat and poultry must be cooked right through.
- Reheated food should be taken to at least 70 °C.
- Food may be reheated in a microwave—take care to ensure that the centre of the food is well heated.
- Liquids should have reached boiling point.
- Store all cooked food at below 5 °C within 1.5 hours of cooking. Never keep cooked foods outside the fridge/freezer for more than 2 hours.
- Thaw food slowly.
- Never refreeze food after thawing.
- Bacterial multiplication occurs between 10 and 62.8 °C.

Transportation
Food should be transported around the hospital on food trolleys, and not in open containers:

- hot food should be transported at over 63 °C;
- cold food should be transported at below 10 °C.

Samples for bacteriological examination
Samples of all prepared foods served to patients should be stored for 48 hours and be available for microbiological investigation in the case of an outbreak of food poisoning. Although this practice is no longer recommended for the UK, it may be useful for other countries.

Cleanliness
Cleanliness is vital in a kitchen:

- No left-over food or raw products should be left out on the kitchen surfaces.
- All drains should be closed or covered with vermin-proof wire mesh.

- All service areas, floors, and surfaces should be washed daily and wiped over (a neutral—pH 7—detergent is preferable).
- All kitchen equipment must be cleaned meticulously (manually or automatically) and stored.
- All spillages must be removed and the affected areas washed.
- The cleaning equipment for each area should be colour-coded and dedicated to that particular area.
- If there is a pest problem, the Pest Control Officer should be informed.

Staff health

- All staff handling food should be screened for stool carriage of Salmonella species and other pathogens before starting to work in the hospital. This should be done via the Occupational Health Department (see p. 170), which should keep a record of every member of staff. A chest X-ray and tuberculin test are also recommended.
- Any diarrhoeal illness, skin infection, or family contact with gastroenteritis should be reported to the Occupational Health Department.
- There should be adequate staff to cope with the workload—staff should not be overworked.
- The work schedules should be planned so that staff do not have to cross from one area to another unless absolutely essential.
- Proper overalls and headgear must be provided. Disposable gloves or food handling tongs and other implements must be provided for those serving food.

Pest control policy

The hospital administration should produce a pest control policy in conjunction with the catering manager and the IC team.

The Pest Control Officer is usually a member of the Estates Management Department and should be contacted immediately if any pests of vermin are sighted in the catering area. He/she should employ a reliable pest control firm, who should respond immediately. A record should be kept of all sightings of pests and vermin.

Cook—chill food

Food prepared using cook—chill methods must be processed according to the strict guidelines available from the Department of Health and HMSO, which lay down the minimum acceptable standards on:

- bacterial colony counts;
- the temperature at which food should be prepared;
- the temperature at which food should be stored;
- the temperature at which food should be served.

Detailed policies are required to ensure that food poisoning outbreaks do not occur. The most common causes of food poisoning are shown in Table 8.1.

Enteral feeds

Enteral feeds are usually available commercially and in-house preparation should be done with care:

- the containers for the feeds should be sterile;
- the feeds should be prepared as near to the time of delivery as possible (feeds should not be stored at room temperature for more than 6 hours);
- fresh feeds should be made for each meal;
- the nasogastric feeding tubes should be rinsed through with sterile water after each feed.

Disposal of kitchen waste

One person should be responsible for the disposal of kitchen waste, and should ensure that all waste is kept in clean, closed containers ready for collection. Cooked food from the wards should be disposed of in macerator units. Although the sale of food or swill is no longer recommended, if the left-over food is fresh, it can be consumed within 12 hours of preparation. In countries where there is a problem of disposal, the left-over food can be buried.

Inspection

Inspection of the premises and catering practice may be carried out *ad hoc* or on a regular basis by the Environmental Health Officer,

Table 8.1 Organisms causing food poisoning

Organism	Food affected	Method of spread	Incubation period (hours)	Method of poisoning
Salmonella	Poultry, meat, eggs	Hands, surfaces, raw to cooked food	12–36	Multiplication of bacteria
Clostridium perfringens	raw meat, soil, dehydrated products, excreta	Spores activated by cooking	22–24	Toxin produced during sporulation
Staphylococcus aureus	Milk, cream, other dairy products	Hands and nose to food	1–6	Toxin not destroyed by heat
Bacillus cereus	Cereals, rice, soil	Inadequate re-heating, moist storage	1–16	Multiplication of bacteria
Campylobacter	Poultry, meat, water, birds, dogs	Inadequate cooking temperatures, careless handling	1–10 days	Multiplication of bacteria

the Pest Control Officer, and the Hygiene Inspection team (made up of the IC doctor, the IC administrator, and the Catering Manager). Any recommendations made by these people should be complied with.

Building and engineering department

The IC team should have an input into:

- the building, planning, or upgrading of the hospital;
- the planning and building of high dependency units;
- the water supply (including complying with the necessary testing for *Legionella* species);
- maintenance of sterilization and disinfection equipment;
- installation of wash-hand facilities;
- planning and maintenance of air delivery units;
- layout and maintenance of the kitchens.

Planning

All building plans must be seen and approved by the IC team, who should ensure that:

- Drains and sewage pipes are sited along corridors or passages and must not run directly above any high risk or aseptic areas.
- Fresh water pipes do not run beside sewage or effluent pipes.
- Fresh water pipes are placed away from sources of excessive heat.
- There is an adequate number of wash-hand facilities, which should be accompanied by wall-mounted disinfectants, paper towels holders, etc.
- All equipment is of a high standard.
- There are proper maintenance contracts for the equipment.
- There is enough space in the ward or cubicle for a patient trolley and for the necessary non-clinical equipment, bed and bed-locker.
- The windows, doors, and other air inlet areas are not be exposed to building dust or excessive street dust, which might cause problems with fungal spores, e.g. *Aspergillus*.

- Lift shafts and service hoists are designed so that air is not sucked back into them.
- All the walls in the operating theatres and high dependency units are covered with an impervious, washable paint, which will withstand frequent washing and cleaning.
- Ceilings are properly insulated and lined with an impervious layer if services are laid along them, so that any leakage damage is kept to the minimum.
- Carpets, if fitted, are washable and can be steam-cleaned.
- Toilet and shower facilities are adequate for the number of patients.
- Isolation cubicles have integrated toilets and shower facilities.

Water supply and control of *Legionella*

A clean water supply is an essential requirement, without which a hospital cannot function adequately. Most, if not all, of the infection control measures in hospitals demand water in one form or another. If there are no defined criteria for hospital water supplies, then the safety standards for drinking water should be applied to all water.

The water supply in some countries may be unreliable, interrupted or contaminated. Contamination often occurs:

- in corroded, old, or leaking pipes;
- when water pipes run parallel to sewage pipes and are contaminated by leakage of effluent;
- within the pipework and delivery system in the hospital.

Water purification is an expensive and difficult undertaking for a hospital and a clean water supply and delivery system should be guaranteed by the authorities. Water is often supplied by the municipal water authorities and is then stored before distribution through the hospital. Such stored water must be monitored for contamination at regular intervals.

In some countries, waste water and sewage from the hospital flows directly into sewers or into open water system, which run into lakes and rivers. Such effluent is usually untreated and is a potential source of endemic waterborne infections. While treatment of effluent is expensive, it should be given serious consideration.

Methods of water purification

A clean water supply cannot be replaced by the following purification methods, which are suitable only for small amounts of water.

Chlorination

Specialist advice should always be sought before deciding on chlorination as the method of water purification:

- Chlorination of individual tanks is possible in small units but is too expensive for a whole hospital. Chlorine at 0.5 p.p.m. for 1 hour will purify river water (30 minutes is enough for well or borehole water).
- Chlorinated water should be dechlorinated prior to distribution because chlorine is corrosive and may damage metal pipework. The water should be dechlorinated to 0.2–0.5 mg/litre of free residual chlorine using sodium thiosulphate or sulphur dioxide (50 g/500 litre water).
- If chlorination is used, the purification system should be tested regularly to ensure adequate chlorine levels.

Filtration

Filtering is extremely expensive and is not cost-effective when dealing with large volumes of water. It is appropriate for pharmaceutical preparations and for drinking purposes, but the capital outlay is too much for a hospital to undertake on its own.

Boiling

Boiling can be used to purify water for drinking purposes but is not feasible on a large scale. It should be included in the public education programme run in clinics and out-patient departments to combat endemic infections at home.

The use of water in hospitals

Water is used throughout the hospital:

- in all wards and operating theatres for hand-washing
- for steam during the sterilization of equipment;
- for laundry and washing;
- in the catering department;
- in the sterile services department;
- for bathing and washing
- for the disposal of body fluids and excrement;
- for drinking;
- in pharmacy preparations.

Sterile water is required for:

- humidifiers and sterile clinical equipment;
- making intravenous fluids;
- making up enteral feeds;
- immunosuppressed patients.

Table 8.2 suggests alternative water supplies should there be problems with the main supply.

Control of Legionella *on health care premises—1989*

The UK guidelines for the prevention of Legionnaire's disease were issued in 1989. A summary is presented here.

Table 8.2 Alternative water supplies]

Use	Alternative choice
Sterile services	Generate steam by boiling water. Use for autoclaves and washing
Washing equipment	Hot water (60 °C)
Hand washing	70% isopropyl alcohol and sustained-action disinfectant (Hibisol)
Drinking water	Boil water and store in clean containers
Bathing/washing	Heat water (in dedicated containers)
General cleaning	Heat water (in dedicated containers)

Water tanks and storage systems

- Health Technical Memorandum (HTM) 27 recommends 24 hours total on-site storage capacity at roof level. There should be minimum heat gain (BS 6700, section 2). The tank should be well insulated and have a properly fitted cover. Temperatures of 20°C or lower should be maintained. All pipes should be tested at regular intervals.

- Before the tanks are cleaned they should be emptied of water and all visible dirt and debris should be removed manually. A detergent and biocide should be used to clean the tank.

- Hot and cold water systems should be flushed with a calculated chlorine concentration of 50 ± 10 mg/litre (or p.p.m.) and left for 1 hour, after which time the chlorine concentration should be over 30 mg/litre. The process should be repeated if this concentration is not achieved.

- Cold water should be distributed in such a way as to minimize heat gain.

- Hot water systems should be fed by cold tanks, the water should then be heated to 60°C and the circulating temperature should be 50°C. The end water temperature should be no less than 50°C and the outlet should be clearly labelled **DANGER! HOT WATER.**

- Hot and cold water pipes should be separated or insulated to minimize heat gain.

- Cold water temperatures should be less than 20°C after running the water for 2 minutes.

- Pipes should be taken from as close to the water draw-off point as possible. For new installations, this should not be more than 300 mm.

- Plastic washers should replace rubber ones.

- Shower heads should be cleaned regularly.

Pools and baths

Hydrotherapy pools, etc. pose no danger of *Legionella* contamination.

Ward closure

If a ward has to be closed for any length of time:

- all taps should be run for 3 minutes;
- the cisterns should be flushed;
- the water system should be disinfected prior to reopening.

Continuous chlorination and routine sampling for *Legionella pneumophila* are not recommended.

Air conditioning systems

- Stagnant or recycled water from the drip tray should not be in the vicinity of air generation.
- There should be no deadlegs or pools of water.
- The circulation pump flow should be able to overcome the resistance of the distribution system and the refrigerated machine condenser.

Disinfectant

- Hypochlorite is recommended as a biocide.
- Protective clothing should be worn when handling hypochlorite.
- Sodium thiosulphate or sulphur dioxide (50 g/500 litre water) is used to dechlorinate the water system.

Laundry

The laundry service is an integral part of the hospital and a regular and clean supply of linen is essential. Many hospitals have problems with the collection and supply and, where a colour-coded system exists but is not implemented, mixed laundry may be sent for cleaning or , even worse, for incineration. A clear policy on the separation, collection, cleaning, and distribution of laundry is important.

Types of laundry

Laundry should be separated into dirty (soiled) and infected linen at ward level. These types should be colour-coded at source.

Laundry collection

In the UK, linen is separated into bags and sent for laundering, but in other countries each item of linen sent to the laundry has to be counted. This requires handling several times:

- Linen should be removed from the bed and counted (tick on a checklist) before being put into the laundry bag.
- Linen should not be soaked or washed on the ward.
- Linen should be sent directly to its destination without any further sorting.

Processing laundry

Dirty linen is treated manually or semi-automatically; infected linen is treated automatically.

Dirty linen—manual processing

Where mechanized systems for dealing with laundry do not exist, laundry is washed by hand:

- Where possible, the dirty linen should be separated using a colour coding system on the ward.
- Laundry should be handled with domestic-types gloves and should be washed at hand-hot temperatures (around 50°C).
- Infected linen should be soaked in extremely hot water before washing.
- The addition of bleach would aids the disinfection process and makes the laundry look fresh.
- Cotton items may be boiled after soaking for 15 minutes.

Infected linen—automated processing

Automatic systems should operate with water at no less than 80°C (up to 85°C) for 3 minutes and have an automated self-loading system that needs minimal handling.

Theatre linen (sterile)

- Theatre linen should be treated apart from other linen.

- Bleach is not recommended for the removal of stains because of fading.
- Theatre linen should be autoclaved prior to use.

Linen for sterile packs, should be treated in the same way as theatre linen.

Education and training

Education and training is one of the most important roles of the IC team. The better the education programme, the better the under-standing and control of cross-infection.

The IC nurse

The IC nurse should be involved with the initial training programme for the trainee nurses and the refresher courses for the senior nursing staff. He/she should be a member of the Nurse Education Management Group.

The IC doctor

The IC doctor should be involved in training medical students, junior medical staff, nurses, and paramedical staff on topics re-lating directly to patient care and management.

The education programme

The education programme may consist of:

- Formal lectures, including an aseptic technique course on hand hygiene, insertion of intravenous cannulae, and urinary catheter-ization.
- Informal teaching sessions, which are used on ward rounds, case discussions, and medical audit meetings. In the UK, medical microbiologists are often involved in advice on antibiotic pre-scribing and can therefore take advantage of this opportunity to discuss aspects of infection control.
- Research projects, which collect data that is presented to the IC

committee. Discussion of the results of such projects with staff is an important part of infection control education. For example:

—After testing the ventilation system in the operating theatre, the method of testing and the implications of the results should be explained to the staff. If any alterations are necessary, discuss the effects of the changes.

—Hand imprints may be taken of staff in a busy intensive treatment unit. The implications of a high carriage of bacteria should be discussed with staff, who should be told the correct techniques for hand-washing and drying. The tests should be repeated on an *ad hoc* basis a month or so later and the improvement that follows improved practice should be pointed out to the staff.

Education needs to be repeated constantly, a fact that can sometimes be discouraging for the IC team, who feel that the message is not getting across. But the ward staff are often overworked and receive a lot of information from many departments. If liaison between the ward the IC team is good, the ward staff will rely on the team for advice when it is needed. For this reason, ward rounds, which emphasize infection control procedures, are important.

Infection control manual

An infection control manual containing all the IC policies and procedures should be available in every hospital area. It is a good educational tool and should be updated regularly.

Monitoring and auditing policies

The basic concepts of the infection control policy should be uniform and tailored to suit units or hospitals as necessary. Monitoring and auditing these policies is a useful educational tool that can be used with all members of staff.

Tools for education

- Slide shows or videos on specific procedures;
- ward rounds with discussion;
- audio tapes of lectures;

Audio-visual aids need not be expensive; they can be produced by amateur enthusiasts or more professionally, by pharmaceutical companies involved in education.

Practical workshops

Workshops involving IC teams from several countries with similar problems and advisors or supervisors from countries with more advanced IC programmes have proved very successful. They are based on discussions of practical problems dealing with the day-to-day practices of infection control. At the end of each session, a policy tailored to the specific requirements of the participating countries is formulated. This type of education helps to produce uniform policies within and between countries. These projects are usually supported by pharmaceutical companies.

Visitors and relatives

Relatives and friends play an important role in patient care in developing countries and the hospital is seen as an extension of the home environment, a view must be respected and that can be used effectively for the benefit of the patient. There are advantages to devolving some patient care to sensible relatives and it is possible to use attentive family and friends very effectively without jeopardizing the principles of infection control. In some cases, if the procedures are explained carefully, the care may excellent (I have seen relatives ventilating a patient with an Ambu-bag for 3 months!). In the UK, open visiting, particularly in the children's ward is becoming increasingly common.

Mothers are the best nurses for their babies and, if well advised, can take excellent care of their children.

Education and training

- Educate one or two members of the family, or friends. Use wall charts, if necessary.
- Explain the infection control procedure simply and clearly and make sure that they understand what is required of them.
- Explain that the patient is at risk from:
  —contaminated hands—it is therefore important that visitors always wash their hands before and after handling the patient;

—poorly prepared or contaminated food;
—visitors with infections;
—relatives of other patients;
—children who do not understand the gravity of infection control.

- Allow a maximum of two visitors at a time—the patient will need to rest and cannot do this if constantly surrounded by a large number of people.

- Explain that there is a risk to visitors, especially children, from the hospital and other patients.

- Give close relatives a duty rota of 2–4 hours each. Let them help.

Relatives and friends can help by:

- Giving the patient a bedpan or urinal when needed (they should be instructed to wash their hands after this).

- Washing and bathing the patient and tending to their toilet.

- Turning the patient in bed (as instructed) and tending to their pressure points.

- Feeding the patient.

- Informing the staff if dressings become soiled.

- Informing staff if the i.v. fluids run through.

- Ensuring that oral medication and i.v. administration are given on time.

Policy for relatives

Relatives attending a patient should:

- Bathe and change into clean clothes before coming to the hospital.

- Wash and dry their hands thoroughly and use an alcohol rub, if provided, before and after touching the patient (for any reason) and after a dirty procedure.

- Avoid touching i.v. sites, urinary catheters, tracheostomy tubes, etc.

- Dispose of waste in the waste disposal unit (and not in the wash hand basins). Left-over food should be disposed of in the waste bin in the kitchen and dishes should be washed in the kitchen.

- Use only equipment and bedding provided by the hospital.
- Avoid touching other patients (and avoid sitting on other patients' beds).
- It is particularly important that relatives and children do not move from one patient to the next.

Food
- no uncooked food should be brought into the hospital;
- all fruit should be peeled;
- the patient should be given only hot food (no cold food or desserts);
- food should not be shared amongst patients;
- relatives should feed only 'their' patient;
- crockery and cutlery should be washed thoroughly in hot water in the kitchen. It should not be shared among patients.

High dependency nursing and the isolation ward

- The isolation policy must be followed.
- Visitors should wear a plastic apron. This should be changed daily.
- Visitors should wear masks and gloves if required, depending on the patient's diagnosis.
- Gloves must be worn when handling bedpans.

The Occupational Health Department

The Occupational Health Department (OHD) provides a service to all staff working on the premises. Its duty is to ensure that:

- Primary health screening for all staff is carried out either by questionnaire or medical examination.
- The immune status of the staff is up to date.
- Sickness of any nature amongst the staff is documented and reported to a medical officer.

- Pre-employment health checks are completed, including stool clearance samples from the catering staff.
- All inoculation and sharps injuries are reported and documented (see Appendix A for an inoculation accident policy).
- Advice on immunization and vaccination is available.
- All members of staff have a health record, which should be updated regularly.
- Other industrial and work-related injuries and diseases are documented and dealt with.

The IC team should work with the OHD whenever staff are involved in an outbreak of an infectious disease. Regular channels of communication must exist to ensure that everyone is kept informed of any potential risk of infection, either amongst the staff or patients. The OHD is an important link between the staff and the IC Committee and ensures the implementation of IC policies.

Sickness reporting to the OHD

The following must be reported to the OHD:

- all infections among members of staff (suspected or confirmed);
- all contacts with infectious diseases, both inside and outside hospital;
- all accidents and incidents of an injurious nature.

The following categories are particularly important for infection control:

- diarrhoea and vomiting, particularly among the catering staff;
- rashes, boils, and skin conditions;
- persistent sore throat;
- conjunctivitis and other eye infections;
- persistent cough lasting more than 2 weeks.

Immunization

All staff should be offered immunization. The recommendations are:

- rubella, especially for maternity staff;
- polio for all staff;

- tetanus for all staff;
- BCG if the Tine of Mantoux test is negative;
- hepatitis B vaccine for all staff (Appendix A gives an example of a hepatitis B vaccination policy);
- additional vaccination may be offered depending on departmental policy.

It is particularly important that hepatitis B vaccinations should be offered to all staff. If a member of staff declines vaccination, this should be documented.

Procedures on inoculation accidents must be circulated to all staff (see Appendix B).

If an OHD does not exist, the hospital administrator should ensure that proper records are kept, until funds can be found to set up an OHD.

Health and Safety committee

All UK work premises are required by law to have a Health and Safety (H&S) committee. A member of the IC team should attend the H&S committee to advise on the risk to staff from infection, and to report back to the IC committee about H&S policies. Recent UK regulations (Control of Substances Hazardous to Health (COSHH) 1990) require the IC committee to consider alternatives to disinfectants, such as glutaraldehyde (see Appendix B), in the disinfection of fibre optics and to consider how to make endoscopy units safer for staff.

Liaison between the H&S officer and the IC committee is necessary to ensure the correct use and application of:

- protective clothing;
- disinfectants and other toxic substances relating to disinfection or sterilization, i.e. ethylene oxide, glutaraldehyde, phenolics, hydrogen peroxide, iodine, chlorine solutions, and alcohols;
- disposal of waste;
- disposal of sharps;
- protection of patients from clinical and non-clinical equipment;
- protections of staff when dealing with contaminated equipment;
- water supply (and Legionnaire's disease);

- kitchens as a source of infection;
- pest control programme and substances used;
- dangerous substances used in the building that may affect the respiratory system, e.g. asbestos;
- radiation protection and disposal of laboratory waste;
- thermal injuries.

Two infections are notifiable to the H&S officer: hepatitis B inoculation accidents and pulmonary tuberculosis amongst the staff.

Recommendations made by the H&S inspector must be carried out. The inspectors have legal jurisdiction in UK hospitals to ensure that their recommendations are followed. They may inspect the premises at any time and ask for written safety policies for each department. Health care practices must try to comply with the regulations, which apply to everyone—patients, staff and other workers—on the site.

Appendices

Appendix A: Example of a Hepatitis B Vaccination Policy

Serum hepatitis (hepatitis B) can be spread by:

- inoculation with blood or blood products;
- sexual contact;
- contact with other body fluids;
- heavy aerosol dispersion of blood products;
- absorption by mucous membrane (in mouth or eye);
- Contamination by particulates in high-risk procedures;
- contamination of damaged skin (eczema, dermatitis, etc.).

In the UK, hepatitis B is an industrial disease and the Director of Public Health should be notified; cases involving health care personnel should be reported to the Health and Safety Executive.

Prophylaxis

Certain health care personnel are at a higher risk of hepatitis B because of increased exposure to blood or blood products or because of repeated contact with known carriers. Risk weighting factors include:

- where a client group is known to have a high degree of hepatitis carriers;
- where the client group is known to include a large number of chronic carriers;
- where procedures may lead to injury—sharps injuries or assaults;
- where the skin is already damaged;
- where workload is erratic, with a high client turnover;
- lack of awareness in staff and clients of the risks and mode of transfer of the virus;
- when staff have received inadequate training;

- when staff are unfamiliar with the work area and with the patients/clients.

Hepatitis B cannot be totally eliminated and vaccination is one of the courses of action that can protect staff who may be at risk.

ALL HEALTH CARE WORKERS SHOULD OFFERED VACCINATION AGAINST HEPATITIS B

Priority should be given to staff who have begun a course of vaccination and to permanent members of the staffing groups who are in direct contact with patients in the high risk categories.

A course of three doses of vaccine is standard, given i.m. in the upper arm 1 and 6 months apart.

Post-vaccination immune status

Serum should be collected from inoculated staff 3 months after the final dose for measurement of HBV antibodies. Approximately 5 per cent of staff may require a fourth dose 6 months after the third because of a failure to develop HBV antibodies. Staff who do not respond after the fourth dose should be advised (by the IC team or OHD) to establish their Hb 'e' antigen status. If found to be 'e' antigen positive staff should be advised against working in high-risk areas and be checked every six months for the development of 'e' antibodies. If 'e' antibodies have developed they may resume work, but only in low-risk areas.

Antibody testing should be carried out again 5 years after the final dose to ascertain whether a booster vaccine is necessary. The onus is on the member of staff to ensure that they are tested (Fig. 8.1).

Immunization is not compulsory, but should a member of staff decline vaccination, this should be noted on their Occupational Health record.

Inoculation accident policy (Fig. 8.2)

- Wash the site of injury as soon as possible under running and allow free flow of blood.
- Report to the senior nurse manager, who should fill out an accident form and send the member of staff to the Accident and Emergency Department to have their tetanus and hepatitis B immunization status checked.

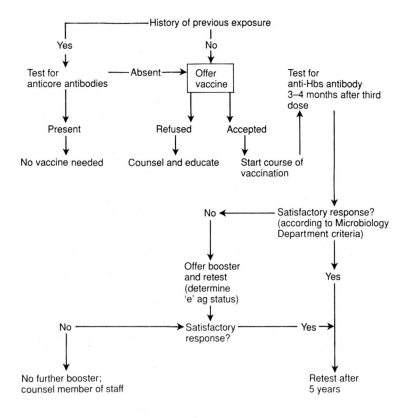

Fig. 1 Hepatitis B immunization policy for staff.

- Take 10 ml blood from the source patient (if known) and from the victim and send to the Microbiology Department for determination of the hepatitis B status of both.
- All blood from staff involved in needle-stick injury should be kept for al least 10 years in case of litigation.

Appendix B: Glutaraldehyde

2 per cent glutaraldehyde is often used in the disinfection of heat-labile equipment. COSHH regulations require its use to be controlled

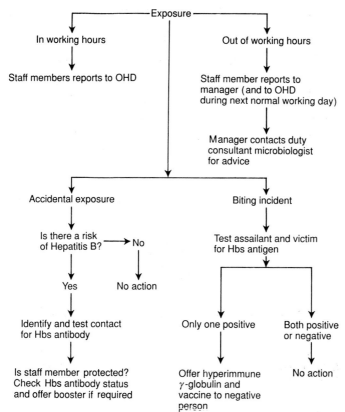

Fig. 2 Hepatitis B accidental exposure protocol.

and the environment rendered safe. The occupational exposure level is 0.2 p.p.m. with 0.82 mg/cm^3 at 25°C (HE. EH40, 1992) time weighted average at 8 hours for aldehyde.

Protective clothing

- Latex or nitrile gloves for handling the equipment;
- eye protection of goggles;
- impervious plastic body covering;
- masks.

Table 1 Inoculation accident and course of action]

Victim	Source	Action to be taken
Immune	Negative or positive	None
Vaccinated but with poor immunity	Negative	Hepatitis B booster
	Positive	Hyperimmune gammaglobulin plus booster
Non-vaccinated	Negative	Start vaccination course
	Positive	Hyperimmune gammaglobulin plus vaccination course

Environment

One of the following facilities should be provided:

- A room with 6–8 changes or air per hour and a local exhaust ventilation system to the outside.

- An extractor or fume cabinet for decanting glutaraldehyde into and out of containers.

- A closed automated system (fibre optic disinfection trolley) .

Extractor cabinets can be fixed or mobile, with a filtration system to remove fumes, however, most of the currently used mobile cabinets do not comply with British Standards.

The environment should be tested by gas chromatography, high performance liquid chromatography or the methyl blue tetrazolium hydrochloride colorimetric method, which tests for the aldehyde group. Testing should be carried out every 14 months. Further test systems are being developed.

Alternatives to glutaraldehyde

At present, no chemical disinfection is more effective than glutaraldehyde:

- Ethylene oxide is an alternative but the initial capital outlay is considerable and this method has to be performed in tightly controlled conditions.

- Quaternary ammonium compounds (QAC) do not kill blood-borne viruses in the time required between endoscopies.

- Alcohol disinfection is possible but the exposure turn-around time is inadequate and there is some evidence to suggest that alcohol can fix viruses.

- A new agent—Virkon—has been introduced recently, but is thought to be less effective than gluteraldehyde against *Mycobacterium tuberculosis* and enteroviruses.

- Pasteurization is a possible alternative but takes too long to be practical for an endoscopy unit, unless there are sufficient endoscopes.

- New chemicals disinfection such as hydrogen peroxide and peracetic acid are currently under investigation.

Glossary

barrier nursing: an obsolete term used to describe isolation facilities, it literally means creating a barrier between the infected patient and hospital staff

carrier state: the presence of a recognized pathogen in a patient or member of staff who does not show any outward manifestation of disease. the pathogen may be transmitted to others and lead in infection

cohort isolation: housing a group of patients carrying the same infecting organism in one ward for isolation purposes

colonization: the presence and multiplication of organisms in body tissue without host response

disinfection: the destruction of micro-organisms, but not usually of spores. The process does not kill all micro-organisms but reduces them to a level that is not usually harmful to health

endemic: a frequently isolated pathogen, which has, essentially, become part of the hospital flora

epidemic: a sudden and dramatic increase in the frequency of isolation of a particular strain of pathogen and/or of an antibiotic sensitivity pattern

hospital-acquired infection: an infection contracted by a patient in hospital. Characterized by the isolation of a known pathogen two or more days after being admitted to hospital

host response: the response shown by an infected individual to the infection, usually pyrexia, raised white cell count, localized erythema, and pain, although not all these may be present

infection: the presence and multiplication of organisms in the body. It is associated with a host response, usually pyrexia, raised white cell count, localized erythema, and pain, although not all these may be present

isolation: nursing a patient separately, usually in a single cubicle, to reduce cross-infection to, or from, the patient

nosocomial infection: an infection acquired in hospital

outbreak: two or more similar strains of the same bacterial species isolated from a patient or member of staff in one unit or hospital area

pandemic: a widespread increase in the spread of pathogens, nationally and internationally

screening: taking samples from infected patients and staff to establish the extent of colonization and spread of an organism. Used when investigating an outbreak

sharp: anything that can puncture then skin

sterilization: a process intended to destroy or remove all living organisms, including spores

ward closure: a ward is closed when no further admissions are permitted, so as to prevent further spread of infection. Where possible, patients are discharged home. Colonized or infected patients should be isolated, not sent to another ward

ward reopening: after thorough cleaning, the ward is opened to new admissions, not to patients previously present on the infected ward (unless they have been screened and cleared of their carrier state)

References and Further Reading

References

Bisno A.L. & Waldvogel F.A. (Eds.), *Infections associated with indwelling medical devices.* Washington DC: American Society for Microbiology.

Cooke, M. (1988). *Hospital infection control guidance on the control of infection in hospitals.* Prepared by the joint DHSS/PHLS Hospital Infection Working Group. London: DHSS.

Currie, E., & Maynard, A. (1989). *The economics of hospital acquired infection.* Discussion paper 65. York: University of York.

Macfarlane, J.T., Ward, M.J., Banks, D.C., Pilkington, R., & Finch, R.G. (1981). *British Medical Journal, 282,* 1838.

Maki, D.G. (1989). Pathogenesis, prevention, and management of infections due to intravascular devices used for infusion therapy. In A.L. Bisno & F.A. Waldvogel (Eds.), *Infections associated with indwelling medical devices* (pp. 161–179). Washington DC: American Society for Microbiology.

Mehtar, S. (1982). Bacteriological survey of patients undergoing TPN and the effects of an i.v. policy. *British Journal of Intravenous Therapy, 3* (8), 3–11.

Mehtar, S. Drabu, Y.J., & Mayet, F. (1989). Expenses incurred during a 5-week epidemic methicillin-resistant *Staphylococcus aureus* outbreak. *Journal of Hospital Infection, 13,* 199–220.

Mehtar, S., Tsakris, A., Castro, D., & Mayet, F. (1991). The effect of disinfectants on perforated gloves. *Journal of Hospital Infection, 18,* 191–200.

Report of the National Survey of Infection in Hospitals 1980. (1981). *Journal of Hospital Infection, 2,* supplement.

Sacks, T., & McGowan, J.E. (Eds.) (1981). International symposium of control of nosocomial infection. *Review of Infectious Diseases, 3* (4).

Whyte, W. (1991). Operating theatre clothing—a review. *Surgical Infection, 3* (1), 14–17.

Whyte, W., Hamblen, D.L., Kelly, I.G., Hambraeus, A., & Laurell, G. (1990). An investigation of occlusive polyester surgical clothing. *Journal of Hospital Infection, 15,* 363–374.

Further Reading

General Reading

Ayliffe, G. A.J., Collins, B.J., & Taylor, L.J. (1990). *Hospital acquired infection, principles and prevention* (2nd ed.). London: Wright.

Cooke Report. (1988) *Hospital infection control guidance on the control of infection in hospitals*. Joint DHSS/PHLS Hospital Infection Working Group. London: DHSS.

Lowbury, E.J.L., Ayliffe, G.A.J., Geddes, A.M., & Williams, J.D. (Eds.) (1981). *Control of hospital infection: A practical handbook*. London: Chapman and Hall.

Maurer, I.M., (1985). *Hospital hygiene* (3rd ed.). London: Edward Arnold.

Wenzel, R.P. (Ed.) (1987). *Prevention and control of nosocomial infections*. Baltimore: Williams and Wilkins.

Economics of Infection Control

Wenzel, R.P. (Ed.) (1987). *Prevention and control of nosocomial infections*. Baltimore: Williams and Wilkins.

Outbreaks

Casewell, M.W., & Hill, M. (1986). Elimination of nasal carriage of Staphylococcus aureus with mupirocin (pseudomonic acid)—control trial. *Journal of Antimicrobial Chemotherapy, 17*, 365–372.

Duckworth, G. (1990). Revised guidelines for the control of epidemic methicillin-resistant *Staphylococcus aureus*. Report of the combined working party of the Hospital Infection Society and the British Society of Antimicrobial Chemotherapy. *Journal of Hospital Infection, 16*, 351–377.

Antibiotic Usage

Garrod, L.P., Lambert, H.P., & O'Grady, F. (1984). *Antibiotics and chemotherapy* (6th ed.). Edinburgh: Churchill Livingstone.

Kucers, A., & Bennett, M.C.R. (1987). *Use of antibiotics* (4th ed.). London: Heinemann Medical Books.

Disinfection and Sterilization

Central Sterilizing Club (1986). *Sterilization and disinfection of heat-labile equipment.* Working Party Report No. 2.

Central Sterilizing Club (1986) *Washer/disinfector machines.* Working Party Report No. 1.

Department of Health and Social Security (1980). *Health Technical Memorandum 10.* London: HMSO.

Gardner, J.F. & Peel, M.M. (1991). *Introduction to sterilization and disinfection.* London: Churchill Livingstone.

HMSO (1989). *Guide to good manufacturing practice for National Health Service Sterile Services Departments (1989).* London: HMSO.

HMSO (1990). *Further evaluation of transportable steam sterilizers for unwrapped instruments and utensils.* London: HMSO.

Blood-borne Diseases

Advisory Committee on Dangerous Pathogens (1990). *HIV—the causative agent of AIDS and related conditions.* Second revision of guidelines. London: HMSO.

British Standard Institute (1989). *Draft British Standards Specification for sharps containers 89/5277.* May 1989. London: BSI.

British Medical Association (1990). *Code of practice for safe use and disposal of sharps.* London: BMA.

Center for Disease Control (1989). *Guidelines for the prevention of transmission of HIV and HBV to health care and public safety workers.* Morbidity and Mortality Weekly Report 38S-6. Atlanta: CDC.

Department of the Environment (1983). *Waste management.* Paper No. 25. London: HMSO.

HMSO (1990) *Guidance to health care workers: Protection against infection with HIV and hepatitis virus.* Recommendations of the Expert Advisory Group on AIDS. London: HMSO.

Health and Safety Commission (1982). *The safe disposal of clinical waste.* London: HMSO.

HMSO (1974) *Health and Safety at Work Act 1974.* London: HMSO.

Hospital Waste Disposal

Johnson, C.D., Evans, R., Shanson, D., Wastell, C. (1980). Attitudes of operating theatre staff to inoculation risk cases. *British Medical Journal of Surgery*, 26 (2), 195–197.

Nelson, S. (1987). Infectious hospital waste: A troublesome costly problem. *Modern Healthcare*, 17, 44.

Royal College of Nursing (1986). *Nursing guidelines on the management of patients in hospital and the community suffering from AIDS* (2nd ed.). London: RCN.

Taylor, L.J. (1988). Segregation, collection and disposal of hospital laundry and waste. *Journal of Hospital Infection, supplement A*, 57–63.

Department of the Environment (1991). *Environmental Protection Act: Waste Management—Duty of care. Code of practice.* December 1991.

Investigation of Infection

Cheesbrough, M. (1984). *Medical laboratory manual for tropical countries, vol. 2. Microbiology. Tropical Health Technology.* London.

Shanson, D.C. (1989). *Microbiology in clinical practice* (2nd ed.). Wright. London.

Recycling of Equipment

Re-use of sterile single use and disposable equipment in the NHS (1986). Proceedings from a conference held 2–3 December 1985 at the Royal Institute of British Architects, London.

US Code of Federal Regulations CRF 21, Part 820. Good Manufacturing practice for medical devices. July 1978.

Operating Theatres

Department of health (1992). *Health Building Note 26. Operating department.* London, NHS Estates.

Hambraeus, A., Laurell, G. (1980). Protection of the patient in the operating suite. *Journal of Hospital Infection*, 1, 15–33.

Lidwell, O.M., Lowbury, E.J.L., Whyte, W., Blowers, R., Stanley, S.J., & Lowe, D. (1982). *British Medical Journal*, 285, 10–14.

Medical Research Council (1962). Design and ventilation or operating suites. *Lancet, ii,* 943.

Catering

Department of Health. Health building note 10. Catering departments. London: HMSO.

Department of Health and Social Security (1987). *Health service catering hygiene.* London: HMSO.

HMSO (1984). *Food Act 1984, C8 30.* London: HMSO.

Occupational Health Departments

Department of Health (1989) *Control of substances hazardous to health. Guidance for the initial assessment in hospitals.* London: HMSO.

Health and Safety Executive Committee (1989). Health and Safety Executive Occupation Exposure Limits. Guidance Note EH 40/ 89. London: HMSO.

Water

HMSO (1989). *The control of Legionella in health care premises. A code of practice.* London: HMSO.

Index